On Being a

DOCTOR

3

On Being a
DOCTOR

3

Edited by
Christine Laine, MD, MPH
Michael A. LaCombe, MD, MACP

AMERICAN COLLEGE OF PHYSICIANS
PHILADEPHIA

Director, Editorial Production: Linda Drumheller
Associate Publisher and Manager, Books Publishing: Tom Hartman
Production Supervisor: Allan S. Kleinberg
Publishing Coordinator: Angela Gabella
Cover Design: Flatiron Industries
Interior Design: Michael Ripca
Composition: Wendy Smith and Michael Ripca

Dust jacket photograph courtesy of Robert Mendle, MD

All selections and photographs in this book originally appeared in *Annals of Internal Medicine*, published by the American College of Physicians.

Composition by ACP Graphic Services
Printing/binding by R.R. Donnelley
Printed in the United States of America

ISBN: 978-1-930513-88-4

07 08 09 10 11 / 9 8 7 6 5 4 3 2 1

Preface

Whether you are doctor, patient, or lover of literature, read this book. In it you will find a collection of stories, essays, and poems that originally appeared in *Annals of Internal Medicine* from 1999 to 2006. One of the world's leading medical journals, *Annals* has published this material for well over a decade in its sections "Ad Libitum," "On Being a Doctor," and "On Being a Patient." The juxtaposition of literature and science in the journal does not concern our readers; in fact, many say that they read these sections before delving into the scientific content. Some readers confide that the literary material is the only part of the journal that they always read. Non-physician family members and colleagues of readers have told us that they turn to these sections whenever they encounter an *Annals* issue in the stack of daily mail. The success of the two previous compilations in this series (1995 and 2000), perennial ACP best-sellers, attests to this popularity. *On Being a Doctor 3* offers a fine sampling of favorite recent pieces.

Why is it that stories about illness and physicians attract such an eager audience? One reason is that diagnosing and treating disease often contains elements of high drama. Second, an aura of mystery often still surrounds the medical profession, the long years of rigorous training initiating us in healing secrets unknown to outsiders. In addition, whether a person has been ill, is ill, or simply fears future illness, there is some comfort in hearing about how others deal with the experience and in gaining insight into the minds of those who care for the sick. Lastly, many doctors themselves are wonderful storytellers.

The frustrations of practicing medicine often overwhelm the many satisfactions of caring for patients. Doctors struggle to navigate the impersonal bureaucracy that health care has become. The public is increasingly disillusioned with the expenses of being sick and doctors who seem to have little time to talk to them. Despite remarkable advances in medical science, many people remain without access to even the most basic health care. On the other side, the financial and personal costs of becoming a doctor continue to rise as the financial and personal rewards sink below other, less noble professions. Reading these stories will help you see why, despite these challenges, most doctors would not dream of doing anything else. And, if you are one of these beleaguered doctors, reading this book will reinvigorate you.

The selections in *On Being a Doctor 3* cover many themes. Because death and dying is the topic that prompts most of the stories and poems that we receive at Annals, many of the pieces herein fall under that topic. Doctors also write movingly about learning and teaching medicine, about aging, and about relating to their patients. In other pieces, doctors tell about the (often dysfunctional, sometimes wonderful) places and systems in which they work and share their observations of the (often dysfunctional, sometimes wonderful) world we live in. Many pieces are terribly sad: "The Cost of Medicine," "Precious Cargo," "A Good Pair of Hands," and "The Pirates," for instance. Some are joyous: "Simple Gifts," "Pretzels and Fruitcake," and "Blue Light and Milk." Others are eerie: "Pronouncing," "The Sharer," and "Homeless." Some are ironic or humorous: "A Tale of Two Patients" and "Foreign Body of the Heart." All are memorable.

Few readers, we are sure, will finish this book without being inspired, appalled, haunted, and deeply touched by many of the pieces found here. Some readers may even be compelled to begin writing themselves. If so, we know of at least one medical journal that would be happy to consider your work.

Christine Laine, MD, MPH
Michael A. LaCombe, MD, MACP

Acknowledgments

How is it that poems, essays, and stories are to be found in an esteemed medical journal? Through the vision of fine editors, three sections comprising this literary material, "On Being a Doctor," "On Being a Patient," and "Ad Libitum," have been part of *Annals of Internal Medicine* for the past 15 years. We thank Bob and Suzanne Fletcher, Frank Davidoff, and Hal Sox for that vision.

Nicole Briglia and Mary Beth Schaeffer do an amazing job shepherding manuscripts through the *Annals* submission, review, and production processes. Without their able assistance, the initial publication of these pieces (and thus this book!) would not have been possible.

For their enthusiastic and unqualified support of this endeavor, we are grateful to Diane McCabe, Bob Spanier, Linda Drumheller, Nancy Matthews, and Steve Weinberger. Many thanks to Tom Hartman for his assistance during the final stages of book production.

Finally, we must thank the photographers who generously gave permission for their work to be used herein: Robert Mendle, MD (dust jacket); Curtis N. Sessler, MD (p 1); Masahiko Ishikawa, MD (p 43); Daniel Jackson, MD (p 89); P. Kahler Hench, MD (p 135); Maureen Beitler (p 171), Jeffrey Levine, MD (p 225); Saul Weinberg, MD (p 249); and Richard Babb, MD (p 323). All of these photographs originally appeared in *Annals*.

Contents

On Being a Patient

Balancing the Personal and Professional

Those Who Are Our Patients

On Aging

On Death and Dying

Hospitals, Health Systems, Contentions

On Society and
the World Around Us

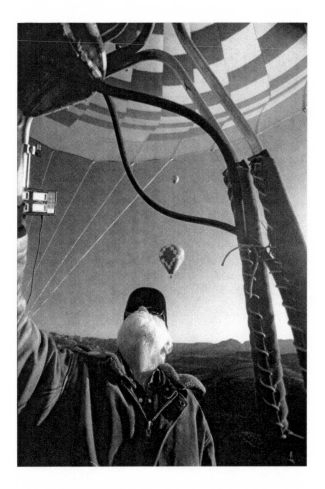

The Pirates

CAMPION QUINN, MD

The two boys jumped from bed to bed, as the ceiling fan creaked and spun lazily through the humid September air. At the height of their leaps, the blades narrowly missed their heads. Liam cried to Martin, "Jump any higher and the fan will cut your head off."

"I'm not scared."

"Me neither, nothing can hurt me," said Liam.

Martin, the taller of the two boys, drew from his belt the ruler that was his cutlass this hot afternoon. He lunged after Liam, thrusting and slashing, chasing him across the stained brown carpet and down the stairs. As he ran through the kitchen, Liam grabbed a wooden spoon from the counter top. This martial parity brought a renewed ardor for the fight. Liam spun and faced his adversary, a duel to the death. Parrying and thrusting, he slashed across Martin's wrist and the ruler fell. With his enemy disarmed, Liam pushed the spoon handle into Martin's abdomen. Falling to his knees, Martin cried, "Arggh, ya got me, Captain Kidd, all the treasure is yours."

"What about the parrot?" Liam asked.

"You can have the parrot too!"

"I guess I'll need a map to find your treasure," suggested Liam.

In search of a treasure map, they headed, at a dead run, for the kitchen table. The battle and the fatal wound forgotten, the buccaneers ripped pages from a school notebook and began to draw maps. Their heads bent in concentration, they created several copies of a treasure map. Each succeeding version contained a different combination of palm trees, Jolly Rogers, dotted lines, and treasure chests. Each chest burst with gems, doubloons, and strands of pearls.

They drew maps, pirates, and galleons for more than an hour, intermittently making sorties to the refrigerator for milk, cookies, and apples. The boys ate noisily and laughed as apple juice dripped from their mouths and chins.

Out in the back yard, they searched for their buried treasure in the pine grove. The needles were dry, and the ground was soft. They began to run, then roll, on the cushion of needles. They tossed pine cone hand grenades at one another from behind the trees, supplying the sounds of the explosions and cries of the wounded. They rolled down an embankment and onto the bottom of a dry riverbed. As they lay on their backs, gasping from exertion, they stared at the deep blue sky, framed by the swaying tops of the pine trees. They lay and talked for a long while, hearing only their own soft voices and the buzzing of the last of the cicadas in the September heat.

Despite being cousins of similar age, Martin and Liam looked nothing alike. Martin was tall, with a wide dark face and straight snowy teeth. His hair was dark, shiny, and uneven on one side where his mother had slipped with the clippers. Liam was thin and fair, with sharp features and golden hair. His front teeth had been missing since the beginning of the summer. This bothered him not a bit. In fact, Liam enjoyed the novelty, and often entertained his friends at school cafeteria by squirting milk through the spaces between his teeth.

"We should be getting back." Martin said. "My Mom'll be home soon, and I've got to finish that math homework."

"Yeah, I guess," said Liam glumly.

Ambling back to the house, they tossed more pine cones, and a branch became a machine gun, which chattered away in the shady pine grove.

In the house, Martin ran upstairs to look for his schoolbooks amidst the bedroom clutter. Liam put away milk containers and swept cookie crumbs off the table with his hand. As he cleaned, he heard his named being called from upstairs. He entered the bedroom, where earlier boarding parties from his cousin's ship had crossed to his. Now he watched his cousin sitting on the edge of his bed, aiming a handgun out the window. The gun was large in Martin's tiny hands, all heavy lines and sharp angles. Its weight, color, and geometry all fascinated him. The gun was cool to Martin's touch, and the oily surface made it difficult for him to grip the gun firmly. The two boys stared, mesmerized.

"Wow, where'd you get that?" Liam finally said.

"From my Dad's closet," Martin confided.

"Why's he have it?"

"Burglars!" Martin said.

Liam was incredulous. "Burglars! You've got burglars?" His tone implied that burglars might be an infestation, like rodents or cockroaches. Liam's eyes quickly scanned the room, as if a burglar might jump out at them from the closet, or from under a bed.

"Nah. Well, I've never seen them, anyway," Martin confessed.

"Then why does he have it?" Liam persisted.

"I guess my Dad thinks it's cool," Martin said.

Eyeing the gun enviously, Liam asked, "Can I see it?"

"Sure, but be careful."

As the gun was passed between their tiny hands, a loud report shattered the silence of the afternoon. Martin, frightened by the noise, dropped the gun. He quickly looked out the window. In his mind's eye, he could see his mother, frantic, racing for the front door. He could easily imagine the beating he would get. He was relieved when he saw no immediate danger, and quickly bent to pick up the gun, intending to wrap it in the oily rag he'd found it in and to put it back on the floor of his father's closet.

It was then that he saw his cousin, lying still on the floor. Below his chin was a small black hole. Blood ran from it and mixed with the golden hair and ended in another dark stain on the carpet. Liam stared blankly at the ceiling fan as it slowly cut the humid September air.

The Red-Pigment Factory

CHARLES WOERNLE, MD

The yellow smoke rises from a multitude of stacks
And delivers to the valley the notice of its source.

Beneath the smoke the ground and all it holds
Lie red, red from the stuff men spend their lives scurrying to form.

Twisted metal and acid liquor give birth to powder Scarlet,
Who flows and spills and fills some bags—and other things besides.

Onto the walls, onto the men, and into their skin it goes,
Carried by the wind that blows the sound of the whistle that rules
their lives.

What Happened in Laramie

DANIEL S. KLEIN, MD

Matthew Shepard was found tied to a fence on the prairie east of Laramie, Wyoming, unconscious after a brutal beating. He died several days later without having regained consciousness.

It was strange and disorienting for those of us in Laramie to be the focus of intense national publicity. For a while, we eclipsed the president and Kosovo as the top news story. News trucks were rolling down the streets, looking for people to interview. A friend from New York called to say that my wife was on national television; a crew had recorded the church service where she had sung. Tom Brokaw in the emergency department, reporters in Burger King.

Here in Laramie, we nurture the belief that we reside in a small, supportive, protective community, shielded from the random violence of urban areas. But this was the third savage murder in a year, each one tearing the community apart in its own way. Just a year ago, the nude body of a 15-year-old girl was found in the hills east of town, with 17 stab wounds. The man who was arrested and convicted was a long-time area resident; acquaintances could not believe he was capable of such horror. Then, in the spring, a 7-year-old child from Laramie who had been visiting family in northern Wyoming was abducted, assaulted, and murdered. Her body was found in a garbage dump. A man with a history of pedophilia was arrested. He pleaded guilty.

And now—the murder of Matthew Shepard. Matt, an undergraduate at the University of Wyoming, was apparently tortured before being savagely murdered. He was tied to a fence and left to die. Many people likened his torture and death to a crucifixion.

The national press made a great issue of the fact that Matt was gay and that his assailants had lured him out of a bar and to his death. He had allegedly propositioned his assailants, which seemed to have triggered their rage. We had thought that our cultural environment tolerated diversity, but people in the gay community tell me that they were exceedingly fearful even before this tragedy, and my children, who have gone to high school and college in Laramie, tell me that gay bashing is common.

Matt was found in an area where I sometimes jog or bike. The press noted with a certain moral smugness that this area was near expensive new homes and that Matt's assailants came from the less wealthy west side of Laramie, somehow implying an issue of class as well as sexual orientation.

The prairie east of Laramie is interesting. From town, it appears to rise as a smooth progression, gaining about 1600 feet of elevation above our high mountain valley. However, after one starts up the incline, the prairie breaks up into a series of rugged canyons that are carved into the hills. Eagles' nests can be found at some of the higher elevations. People who live close to the prairie keep their dogs in at night for fear of mountain lions. My dog and I have been stalked by coyotes several times. The increase in elevation is associated with a dramatic change in climate, from high desert near town to forest upland. It is an inspiring landscape, an area of overwhelming beauty.

The University of Wyoming, for residents of the state, has one of the lowest tuitions of any university in the country, and it is possible, if not easy, for Laramie residents to earn enough to put themselves through school. This nurtures another of our cherished beliefs here, that we do not have a compartmentalized community.

I never met Matthew Shepard, nor his alleged assailants. Nevertheless, his death has affected me profoundly. It was a blow to my perception of my community. However, the crisis was much more than a mere philosophical abstraction. On the Thursday morning that Matt was found, I stopped by the emergency department after my hospital rounds to see whether there were any patients that I needed to know about. The emergency department physician remarked that he had treated some kids who had assaulted each other; he had sent two of them to Fort Collins for neurosurgical care. There seemed, as I understood the story then, to have been a bar brawl in which alcohol or drugs—unfortunate byproducts of college towns—had played a part, and my colleague and I commiserated with each other that the trouble our teenage kids got into was minor by comparison. That afternoon, the local newspaper, the *Laramie Boomerang*, had a brief story, without details. The incident still seemed relatively innocent.

The next day, the crime, in its enormity, was reported in the paper and quickly picked up by the wire services. It was national news by evening. A police officer called me to ask me to consult in my role as county health officer, telling me that some of the responders at the scene had been exposed to Matt's blood and inquiring whether there were any concerns about infectious disease. The public health officer in rural Wyoming has no staff or budget, and hours of my time were involved in mobilizing the state health department to assist us. Because I also serve as the medical director of the jail's health clinic, the medical needs of the alleged assailants were brought to my attention.

I discussed the crisis with my daughter at dinner. She is a first-year student at the university and had attended Laramie High School. She knew one of the alleged assailants fairly well and was surprised that he was implicated. She felt that students were not sympathetic to gays but couldn't understand how the crime had happened.

Finally, five days after the crime, I got a phone call from one of my patients, a 75-year-old woman with severe congestive heart failure. Her only child, a daughter, had died in the hospital of complications during what was expected to be a routine surgical procedure, and that woman's son—my patient's only grandson—was in jail accused of the murder. She could not believe it. He had always been such a good boy; they had always been such pals; he always did all he could to help out his grandparents; he had friends who were gay. She said that he was the only grandchild she would ever have. Here was a grieving grandmother's sad effort to make sense of the tragedy but also an opinion different from that of the press, which had demonized the alleged assailants. Indeed, the other alleged assailant had been an Eagle Scout, and acquaintances of his spoke publicly of their surprise and disbelief.

A series of community vigils followed, many extensively reported in the national press. Somehow, the intrusiveness of the press vulgarized a profoundly disturbing personal and local event. All at once, each speaker at each rally was speaking to a national audience as well as to those of us who shivered in the cool evening trying to express our sadness and find our way.

There have been no allegations of conspiracy. In some ways, it would have been easier if the incident were an orchestrated campaign of Aryan Nation. Then we could have had a villain to blame. Instead, we have the paradox of kids who seemed to be making it despite hardship but suddenly felt a rage so terrible that it consumed them—the paradox of ordinary people who commit extraordinary crimes. A prominent pastoral leader of the community admonished everyone to look within themselves for the seeds of intolerance. How many racial, gender, or ethnic slurs do we let slip by because it is too awkward to challenge them? Do we all have within us the capacity to commit crimes as violent as this? Can we say that murderers are somehow different from ordinary people, or do ordinary people have the ability to lose control and become murderers?

This afternoon, I went for a run on the prairie east of town and my route took me close to the fence where Matthew was left to die. The late afternoon autumn light in the canyons and hills was incredibly beautiful. The peace, solitude, and solace of the prairie were overwhelming. The violence of natural forces that had created this landscape was somehow more understandable than the human violence that had corrupted it.

Madrid, March 11, 2004

ALICE GIFFORD

How have you broken into my heart
All you who have gone?
Who never said goodbye,
Nor adios nor adieu
Nor any other farewell
To those you loved,
Nor said "Look after the children"
Or its equivalent in any language,
But simply went torn and shoeless
Into the heavens,
While those who sent you dreamed of Paradise.

Innocent

H. JOAN WAITKEVICZ, MD

I came to South Florida from an urban medical practice in the North. Three years later, I am still surprised by many things. Mango trees, royal palms, egrets, ibises, and pelicans are commonplace. A fly-by of squawking green parrots is a treat.

One big difference is how my neighbors experience poverty. Here, people who don't have a car are poor in a way that could not be imagined in New York City. You have to wait until a neighbor can drive you for your food, toiletries, medical visits, anything at all. Or, in 80- to 90-degree weather, you must walk or bicycle a long way, or wait at the bus stop without shade. If there is nobody to watch your children, you bring them with you. You try not to leave them home alone.

My friends and I volunteer as escorts at a women's health center. This is necessary because, every Saturday morning, antiabortion protesters stand outside the clinic for 2 or 3 hours. Some pray. Some hold signs. Even in the heat, some hold their young children instead of signs.

When a patient pulls into the center's driveway, some of the protesters walk up to the car, videotape her or her driver, and try to talk them out of coming in. They continue to call out to the patient as she walks from her car to the front door.

We are not supposed to confront the protesters. We stay in the parking lot, offer to walk with the patient, and be a quiet, reassuring presence until she is inside the door. If she is having an abortion, someone will be there to wait for her, a friend, spouse, mother, sister, or grandmother. They may pass the time by talking with us. We talk about our belief in her right to have this abortion, to have some choice in the direction of her life.

The center also pays an off-duty police officer to be there all day for protection. He calls a police officer on duty if there is trouble.

One day last year, Harriet, an experienced escort, saw several protesters surround a young Central American woman who was walking toward the driveway. One was a nun and one appeared to be a priest. Harriet encouraged the woman to enter. The group moved the woman farther down the sidewalk. Harriet went inside and told the staff. Ramona, a Spanish-speaking counselor, came out in her scrub suit and beckoned to the woman.

We waited with Ramona for 15 minutes or more. The woman, still surrounded, appeared upset, but made no move either to come in or to leave. Finally, Ramona called a supervisor and together they walked over to the woman. A protester immediately called the policeman. She filed a complaint that the staff and the "proabortion protesters" had "violated the statute and interfered with [her] counseling."

The woman walked into the parking lot with Ramona. I went up to her to offer encouragement, but Ramona said, "She's not here for an abortion. She has some other problem." They went inside.

I told Harriet, "She wasn't even here for an abortion. That's how much they listened to her."

Harriet called to the nun, "You know, she wasn't even here for an abortion!"

Innocent!

She walked from somewhere, hatless in the sun. She was too polite to turn her back on a priest and nun, however long they spoke with her. She knew she wanted health care and went to considerable trouble to get it.

If she was coming for birth control, perhaps she felt some guilt in front of a priest and nun. But she did not walk away. She stood until Ramona came for her.

She was "innocent" of the battle lines that had been drawn up around her. If she needed birth control, and succeeded in getting it, she might stay that way.

Other women around the world also find someone to watch their children, and travel long distances to get to a clinic that will give them birth control or other reproductive health care.

These clinics have traditionally enjoyed the support of the United States government and the United Nations. When they close, the consequences include more maternal and infant mortality, more unplanned pregnancies, more pregnant girls, more women with HIV infection and other sexually transmitted infections, more unsafe births, and more unsafe abortions.

In January 2001, President George W. Bush re-imposed the "Mexico City rule" on reproductive health programs abroad. President Reagan had instituted the rule in 1984, and President Clinton had rescinded it in 1993. Also known as the "gag rule," it takes away American funding from programs that provide or give referrals for abortions, campaign to legalize abortion, or even discuss abortion with a patient as an option.

In 2002 and 2003, the Bush Administration vetoed the Congressional appropriation for the United Nations Population Fund. Congress has approved a $34 million contribution for 2004; President Bush is reviewing it. It is estimated that our $34 million contribution for the year 2002 could have prevented two million unwanted pregnancies and nearly 800,000 abortions. The consequences of the 2003 shortfall have not yet been calculated.

Charleston Sunset

AMY WEAVER, MD

The same fire,
   which has lit
the edges of the world,
   feeds the glow inside of me
and I am standing
   with a handful of questions.
As I drop them,
   one by one,
you dip behind a boat
   to pick one from the pile at my feet:

How could you end this moment
   in any more splendor?

But, you stay tucked away,
   without a response,
no smoke, no suddenness,
   just a quiet dwindling of a gentle flame,
and, there I am,
   standing empty-handed,
with nothing else left to hold
  … besides my breath.

The Greater Rock of Ages Baptist Church

ANNE L. PETERS, MD

I work in a busy hospital-based clinic, staffed by a large but competent and consistent group of secretaries, nurses, clerks, and other personnel. When the fiancé of one of the scheduling clerks was killed in
an automobile accident, I felt obliged to attend his memorial service.
Betty, the employee, was approximately my age, in her late 30s. Although she sometimes seemed overwhelmed by the needs of scheduling (and rescheduling) our many patients, she was always kind and
helpful. I knew nothing of her personal life but was told that she had
two sons from a previous relationship and had known Jim, her fiancé,
for the past seven years. For an African-American woman struggling
to raise two boys in the Los Angeles area, losing the man who had
served as their father and role model would be a great tragedy. Working as a physician, I have collected people's life tales as I obtain their
medical details. Putting people in their personal context helps me understand how they may internalize the medical advice I dispense. Attending Jim's memorial service provided a large dose of context.

Directions to the service were hurriedly given to me while I was
distracted in a busy clinic. I asked no questions and shoved the piece
of paper into a pocket of my white coat. Two days later, as I pulled out
of my driveway, I tried to decipher where I was going. After searching

through my map book, I realized that I was headed for the heart of Watts, the vast, forbidding, primarily African-American ghetto in south-central Los Angeles. My previous experience with Watts had been limited to driving through it on the freeway (hoping my car wouldn't break down) and watching television footage of burning structures during the various riots that had occurred there. I was unnerved, but I proceeded anyway.

When I turned off the freeway, the streets of Watts looked just as I'd expected: small, aging houses, many liquor stores, and old rusted cars. But what I hadn't expected was that on nearly every block was a small church, a brave beacon of faith in the midst of poverty. I drove past many of these houses of worship until I spotted the one I was seeking, the Greater Rock of Ages Baptist Church.

The church was a small, white, wood-frame structure with few adornments. A crudely made banner hung behind the altar proclaiming, "We love Jesus." A sign on the wall noted that eight people had attended Sunday school the previous week and $3000 in donations for the church had been collected during the past year. A few framed photographs of past and present ministers hung askew around the altar. A large, poster-sized picture of Jim's face, grainy and slightly indistinct, hung down from the front of the podium. Eight rows of hard wooden pews faced the front of the church for those who attended the church services, and two smaller rows of pews were set behind the altar for the choir. There were no religious icons, no statues, no stained-glass windows, no flowers, not even hymnals or Bibles. Just space for the congregation, minister, and choir, with faith, hope, and God to help them endure.

I was a foreigner in this world, and although I was treated graciously I was also kept distant. Two other physicians who worked at the clinic showed up, and we were seated together, off to one side, at the front of the church. Betty later told me that her friends were amazed that "white folks" would venture into their world—amazed and a little dubious about the wisdom of our traveling into Watts.

The service began with songs and prayers and quickly moved on to the period called "Remarks." This was when Jim's friends were asked to talk about him, remembering who he was and what he meant to them. All of the men who spoke knew Jim through the various rehabilitation programs they had attended together. Some had been in prison. They spoke of the bonds they had had with a kind man who could help others but not himself. The women spoke of suffering and urged Betty to be strong. They understood; they had all lost the men in their lives. I wondered how often these church services occurred in this part of town. Much more often, it seemed, than in mine. But the speaker who made me weep was Daryl, Jim's 9-year-old stepson.

Daryl was dressed in a teal suit, a white shirt, and a simple tie. He stood bravely in front of the microphone, his child's voice crackling over the poor-quality public address system. From memory, he recited a speech about his father. He spoke of how he'd hated Jim for always forcing him to do his homework and finish his chores, but how he desperately wanted, now that Jim was gone, to hear his voice again, reminding him to do his tasks. He never faltered as he spoke, despite the tears that were trickling down his cheeks. Under Jim's influence, Daryl had grown from a mediocre student with a bad attitude to an outstanding student who hoped to be accepted into a high school for gifted children. What would happen to Daryl without Jim? Would the lessons learned be enough to help him survive in such a difficult environment, or would he return to his old ways?

After the Remarks, the minister delivered the eulogy. Unlike in other Christian services I have heard, there was no mention of sin and redemption, no sense of judgment. Simply believing in God was sufficient, all that was required to enter into the gates of heaven. Clearly, for this congregation, that message was what was needed to provide comfort and hope. When the minister had finished speaking, the congregation began singing a lively revival tune, swaying and clapping. The three of us in front tried to participate, clapping slightly out of synch although not without a reserved sort of spirit.

I stood in front of the church after the service, watching a variety of people walk and drive by. All African-American, all poor. Most had a sense of tired resignation, some had a spirit of hope despite the despair all around them, and others projected a defiant air of anger. I have known of that anger since I was a little girl.

When I was 5 years old, my grandfather, a newspaper editor from a small Midwestern town, visited my family in New York City during the Harlem race riots. Always a reporter, he wanted to see the riots firsthand. He drove me into Harlem, past the police barricades and into the middle of the burning tenements. He stopped when the car became surrounded by an angry mob of protesters. With terror in his eyes, he told me to duck under the dashboard. The protesters began rocking the car from side to side, threatening to light it on fire. Trapped, my 6-foot 6-inch grandfather did what he always did: He talked to people. He rose from the car and was able to convince the crowd to help us to safety. I didn't hear his words, but I saw the anger on the faces of the African-American men change into a reserved friendliness as the fear left my grandfather's face. The crowd surrounded the car again, this time forming a human shield to lead us out of the ghetto. The protesters scattered as soon as we reached the police, who were stunned and angered by my grandfather's escapade.

Although my grandfather and I decided not to tell my parents about our experience, the images from it remain with me. It created an awareness that was reinforced when I worked in developing countries and in various public hospitals in the United States, an awareness of the rage created by oppression and the enormous capacity for humanity that exists within us all.

I left Jim's memorial service reawakened to the world that exists next to mine, so close and yet almost as far away as Africa. It is important to remember how different our lives can be. It reminds me of how fortunate we are and how much work must be done to help those who have less. I plan to visit the Greater Rock of Ages Baptist Church again next year, on a more cheerful occasion. It is a good place for worship.

Emergency

RONALD A. CARSON, PhD

Most mornings I enter the building that houses my office through the back door. And most mornings my mind is elsewhere. I am preoccupied with thoughts of the day ahead: things to accomplish, people to see, meetings to attend, a lecture to give, deadlines to meet.

But this morning, as I cross through the trauma center garage where I park my car, on the ground floor beneath the helipad, a man approaches me, disheveled, emaciated, his eyes a little wild. He walks straight toward me, quickly. I try to seem nonchalant, but I'm no longer preoccupied with anything but my immediate surroundings. I'm focused. The man has my attention.

When we are within touching distance he stops abruptly, holds out his hand (or is he reaching for me?), and mumbles something I don't quite catch. Directions maybe? People often ask for directions down here. I ask, "What'd you say?" "Can you spare some change?" he repeats, more slowly. And then, as if to assure me he's no panhandler, he thrusts his other arm forward to show me a soiled, makeshift bandage barely concealing a suppurating wound. "I got hurt. Been waitin' to get in. I need to get somethin' to eat," and he gestures toward the vending machines in the bare waiting room just behind us at the top of the ramp. I reach into my pocket and empty what change I have into his good hand and ask, "Will that help?" He replies, with gratitude, I think (his agitated expression doesn't change), "If that's all you can spare." Whereupon he wheels about and retraces his steps jerkily toward the snack machines.

I too turn, and continue to my office. I feel the softness of the leather attaché case tucked under my bare, unspoiled arm. I look down and see my $200 shoes. I notice the oil drippings all over the garage floor from the dilapidated vans and pickups that deliver their damaged human cargo to the ER. I become aware of an acrid odor in the humid morning air. I hear the wail of a siren approaching from afar, and the throbbing beat of the rotor blades of the MEDIVAC helicopter landing on the roof, the air around me pulsating from the downward pressure. And in my mind's eye I see the jail bus, with the bars on the windows, turn the corner toward the clinics. That must have happened as I got out of my car when the intersection was in my line of vision. But I don't remember seeing the bus then; I only see it now.

As I pass out of the garage into the sunlight, I see a morbidly obese woman, her legs swathed in elastic wrappings, leaning hard on her walker, lugging her great weight toward the hospital one labored step at a time. I notice for the first time a sign that's surely been there several years: *We care about your health. Our facilities and grounds are a smoke-free environment.* On the benches beneath the sign the medically dispossessed gather, stealing a smoke, staring down and out, worrying, waiting.

To Be a Doctor in Jerusalem: Life under Threat of Terrorism

YISHAI OFRAN, MD
SHADEN SALAMEH GIRYES, MD

In 1948, when the state of Israel was established, Jerusalem was divided between Israel and Jordan, not through any deep reflective process, but merely because of the positions of the opposing armies at the time. Consequently, Mount Scopus, the location of the Hebrew University campus, established on 1 April 1925, and Hadassah University hospital, became an Israeli enclave in the midst of an Arab population. But a university and a hospital could not function under these conditions. Consequently, they were moved to the western part of the city. Since 1967, however, Israel assumed control of East Jerusalem, and the hospital on Mount Scopus was reopened. The Hebrew University returned to the mountain as well. Still, the surrounding population remained mostly Arab. Today, a hospital in which 90% of the staff is Jewish serves a mostly Arab community.

This article reflects our daily experience as doctors in Hadassah Mount Scopus Hospital. We are two residents—one Jewish, one Arab—working together in the internal medicine ward.

More than two and a half years of terrorism have claimed many victims. Among our hospital staff, an attending physician was murdered on his way home. A pregnant nurse in her ninth month from our ward was ambushed and shot five minutes from her home. Her father was killed, and she was severely wounded. An emergency department nurse triaged her own son, who was wounded in one of the terror attacks on the Ben-Yehuda pedestrian mall. Another nurse lost her daughter to terrorists, and the secretary for the hospital's chief executive officer lost her brother, who was murdered along with his fiancée. Familiarity with so many victims lies as a dark shadow over the hospital.

Our Arab patients have their own share of suffering. Some have had their loved ones injured and their homes demolished. Some have faced difficult delays or were humiliated at military checkpoints. The tension is high, and all of us, caregivers and patients alike, carefully walk a thin line. The vast majority of our patients are not connected to atrocities, but many of them support the Palestinian struggle. Wherever Jews and Arabs live so closely, the conflict affects most aspects of life. The neighborhoods one chooses to live in, the public transportation one uses, the place one goes shopping are all affected by the situation. In almost every aspect of life, people trust and prefer to seek help from people of their own nationality. The hospital is the only place left where Jews and Arabs actually meet.

Dr. Ofran, the Jewish physician: As years go by, my Arabic improves and my conversations with my patients extend to personal issues, sometimes even to politics. More than once I have been told by patients that Jews have no right to live in this country and that I "should return to Europe." One night, as we were in the emergency department treating casualties from a terrorist attack, I overheard a conversation between two young Arab patients in the hallway. In Arabic, they were discussing their anger at the long wait because of the treatment of the terrorists' victims. It was very hard to hear them wishing that all "the Jewish soldiers would die," and it was even harder not to respond.

Dr. Salameh, the Arab physician: I have experienced certain difficulties when treating patients—but in my case, Jewish patients. I'm an Israeli citizen and graduated from medical school in Jerusalem, so I speak Hebrew very well. One day, during morning rounds, one Jewish patient asked for advice: She didn't trust the Arab nurse who passes medications. She preferred, she said, having a Jewish one like "us." I couldn't contain myself. "I am also an Arab!" I said. She was astonished.

Once, during a terrorist attack, I approached a young Jewish patient who was cursing Arabs in general. I wondered what his response would be when he discovered that the doctor who was treating him was one of those he was cursing. On another occasion, a young Jewish patient cursed me and refused my help because he hates Arabs.

Outside the hospital, I face similar difficulties. Whenever a security checkup takes place, Arabs are treated with more suspicion than Jews. Since I have to separate myself from my own feelings and opinions when treating patients, I wonder why the airport workers can't do the same. Why should I be treated as a "suspect" until proven otherwise?

Both physicians: We have been taught to believe that intimacy and frank conversations are beneficial to patients and caregivers. We both experience difficulties with patients because of our nationalities. All over the world, physicians face racism and evil. Terrorism, however, is harder to deal with. Although a racist man can be identified by his behavior, a terrorist may behave as everyone else does. Living under the threat of terror, we find ourselves becoming more suspicious. We search for potential bombers on the buses we take home. We plan our route avoiding dangerous areas.

Suspicion and fear are contrary to intimacy. At the hospital, we mustn't view patients and their relatives as a potential threat. The patient who cursed all the Arabs reminds Dr. Salameh of the difficulties she and other Arabs experience on Jewish streets. Dr. Ofran, like every Jewish man, serves a month annually as a soldier in Israel's reserve force. The patients who wished death for the Jewish soldiers were speaking about him, too. When so many people whom you knew were murdered, it's hard to ignore such thoughts.

At what threshold should an attending physician be called from home? What are the medical conditions that dictate a certain test? There are no clear-cut answers to these questions. The more available the attending, the more he will be called. Similarly, the more available the procedure, the more likely it will be performed. In Hadassah

Mount Scopus, availability is a complicated issue. A significant number of senior doctors, nurses, and technicians live in Jewish settlements in close proximity to the Palestinian Authority. The Palestinian terror groups ambush them on their way from their homes to the hospital. Because of this, a doctor's home address has become a consideration in deciding whether or not to call the doctor on call from home. Despite the danger, physicians, technicians, and nurses come to work every day and never hesitate if they are called at night. But we, as residents on duty, are aware of their imminent danger and factor that in when calling them at home. Our primary obligation is to help the patients, but we are also committed to reducing our colleagues' exposure to danger.

Dr. Salameh: National tensions are beginning to penetrate the walls separating the hospital and the outside world. A nurse who argued with an Arab patient entered the staff room and complained, "They should go to an Arab hospital, not to ours ..."

I responded, "Will your next step be to kick me out of the hospital because I am an Arab doctor?"

"No, no," she said, "it's something else."

Is it?

Dr. Ofran: Patients who share a room may become friends and enjoy each other's company. In order to engender a pleasant atmosphere in the ward, we attempt to match patients according to their age and medical condition. However, in these days of tension, some patients demand a separation between Jews and Arabs. What should be done when a patient or his family want to move to a different room to avoid being with Arabs or Jews? Nurses are guided by myriad considerations. Some are medical (isolation, monitoring, equipment), while others are nursing considerations (distance from bathroom, dementia, age, sex). Clearly, these considerations are primary. It is also clear that segregation of patients based on their nationality must be prevented at all costs. Yet, should all requests of this sort be declined without consideration?

The assignment of patients to the intensive care unit or to a regular ward is based on purely medical considerations. One winter night,

I admitted an Arab patient to the intensive care unit. The Jewish patient who was lying in the next bed rudely expressed his objection to his new neighbor. My attempts to calm him failed, and, having no other option, I demanded that he choose between an Arab neighbor and a regular ward. Regrettably, he decided to move to the regular ward, even though in my view he needed to be in the intensive care unit. What would you have done? How can we change the atmosphere? Is it even possible?

On the afternoon of 11 September 2001, I began my shift. The television sets in the rooms were broadcasting children's programs. The ward was calm. Suddenly all of the channels broke in with the news of the hijacked planes. Doctors, nurses, and patients stared at the television screen in the hallway. From one room, a small and unrepresentative group of four Arab patients exulted, "Bush got it!" How should I have responded? I was extremely angry. How could I keep treating these people appropriately? Understanding, empathy, and a sincere desire to help, which are so important in my contact with patients, had been replaced with anger and scorn. From that moment on, any smile on their faces seemed to be mockery. I was glad that none of them were my personal patients. For their own good, I did not tell their doctor in the morning about this incident.

Many times, I have treated those suspected of committing terrorist attacks and even terrorists who were wounded while committing their crimes. It's easy to concentrate on the suffering of the patients and give them the best treatment possible, even if they are evil, when someone else will decide about their guilt. I find it difficult to deal with situations when I am obligated to remain silent, and I know no one will condemn or punish those who support evil.

Dr. Salameh: I just can't understand how people who suffer can enjoy the suffering of others. I feel anxious about being included in this group just because of shared ethnic origin. It is brutal to enjoy the pain of others and to encourage violence, even in one's thoughts. This behavior is a certain prescription for an unpleasant relationship between two peoples.

Both physicians: The basic infrastructure of terrorism is popular support. It's everyone's duty to protest against any kind of support of terrorism. Physicians should walk a thin line: Condemn all signs of terrorist support on one hand, while showing empathy and understanding on the other. On two occasions, visitors or patients in our department rejoiced when news about a terrorist attack was aired. To prevent these reactions, the nurses usually turn off the public television in the hall whenever terrorist attacks take place.

Hatred and violence in the streets project into the hospital. There have been attacks on ambulances. Twice, a Molotov cocktail was thrown into the yard of the hospital. Despite the violence, despite the relative accessibility of weapons and the nationalistic tension, we remember our oath to help all patients according to their medical conditions alone.

But this is never easy.

Sabir, Patient 4914

JASON STAMM, MD, MAJOR, USAF, MC

"Shukren le linqathi."

"He says, 'Thanks for saving me,'" explains the interpreter as we approach the bedside of patient 4914. His name, which we usually remember to use, is Sabir.* Sabir, the Iraqi policeman who has been with us longer than any other patient in the short history of our facility, is the last patient to be seen on ICU rounds in the Air Force Theater Hospital at Balad Airbase, Iraq. He received a gunshot wound to the abdomen and currently suffers from "abdominal catastrophe," an uncomplicated term to describe a complicated medical and surgical course that has resulted in an open abdomen, limited enteral function, and a dependence on parenteral nutrition. Bed-bound and weighing about 100 pounds, he is not nearly the man he was when he arrived here.

With an awkward feeling of undeserved praise, I ask the interpreter to tell Sabir, "You are welcome," and looking at my notes, begin Sabir's daily presentation to the other physicians of the ICU team. "No significant events in the past 24 hours. Vitals stable. Exam unchanged." I don't have a chance to get to the rest of my brief presenta-

---

*Patient name and identifying number have been changed.

tion before an approaching helicopter, its conversation-deafening and air-reverberating presence easily drowning me out through the tent walls of our hospital, signifies the arrival of yet another trauma victim. We finish rounds on Sabir quickly, examine his abdominal tubes and dressing, write a few orders, and prepare for the arrival of the next patient.

I am a military internist deployed to an expeditionary hospital that cares for injured American and Iraqi military and police personnel. Most patients here have suffered some combination of burn, blast, or penetrating trauma from gunshots or improvised explosive devices. American are treated and removed from the Middle East theater of operations within hours of arrival to our hospital via the medical aero-evacuation system; they leave us with a sense of mission accomplished, perhaps because of assured outcomes at other U.S. hospitals. The relevance of the care we provide to our Iraqi patients, however, is less certain. Iraqi patients usually remain with us for a week or so of stabilizing surgery and ICU care before being transferred to the Iraqi health care system, and we do as much as we can to maximize the long-term chance of success for these patients. We make an effort not to transfer patients until we are confident that the Iraqi medical system can provide adequate care, yet we recognize that medical capabilities in this war-ravaged country are limited. The reality is that the outcome for many of these injured Iraqi soldiers and policemen once they leave our care is uncertain; we rarely learn their fates.

Despite spending more time with our Iraqi patients than we do with our injured American servicemen and women, we are often less familiar with them. Most Iraqi patients arrive at our facility with neither a name nor a background and are assigned a 4-digit identifying number. Sadly, because of injuries, language, and the usual ICU impediments of sedation and mechanical ventilation, many Iraqis are known only by this number during their stay. Patient 4914, Sabir, is an exception to the usual course of Iraqi patients under our care. Sabir has been with us for over 5 months, and his prolonged stay has broken through the common barriers of injury and culture. Many of us, myself included, have come to know Sabir as a person, and his daily presence and the strong feelings that he elicits in those who care for him have made him a fixture of this experience. I have had conversations with Sabir, discovering his past and his personality, and learned that we are the same age. I have even met his family, who travel over dangerous roads to visit him regularly. Through caring for Sabir I have learned a few words of Arabic—"*Alam*" (pain), "*dawa*" (medication), and "*shukren*" (thank you) are often heard from him—and he has learned a smattering of English. Sabir is the most personable Iraqi I have cared for in this often impersonal environment. Unfortunately, our shared knowledge of each other does not transcend the reality of the situation in Iraq. Sabir's inability to tolerate enteral nutrition makes him dependent on our resources. Transfer to the Iraqi health care system, which cannot provide extended parenteral nutrition, would be a death sentence.

Our ICU rounds deliberately end with Sabir every day, ostensibly for infection control purposes, since Sabir is colonized with a multidrug-resistant *Acinetobacter* species. However, he is also the last patient seen every day in unspoken recognition that we struggle to care for him; he requires nearly constant attention. His debilitation and inability to do much for himself, and his abdominal wounds that require frequent assessment of drainage and dressings, are significant nursing issues that are physically demanding and that detract from the ability of the ICU staff to attend to other patients. The healing of patient 4914's abdominal wounds is an arduous process, one that requires frequent trips to the operating room for enteral revision, skin grafting, and drain placement. Separate from the physical burden of his care are the reservations about the therapeutic course we are following. Reluctantly expressed, as if the thoughts should never have entered our consciousness, is the recognition by his American caregivers that patient 4914 consumes a large amount of limited U.S. military medical resources, which are provided via airlift and vehicle convoy through hostile territory for the care of our injured soldiers. In addition, there is a sense of futility to our care, in that the progress of patient 4914 has been slow and troubled by setbacks, such as hospital-acquired pneumonia and catheter-related sepsis. We know he lacks the means by which to leave his home country for care elsewhere, and the care he needs will probably not be available from indigenous resources in Iraq for some time to come. We see in front of us a greatly diminished person, with an open abdomen, tracheostomy, and unnaturally thin arms and legs devoid of muscle mass, who consumes much of our energies, and whose road to recovery, if ever achieved, will be long. We keep patient 4914 alive for the time being with our knowledge and capabilities, but to what end? Will our efforts and use of limited American medical resources ultimately result in a meaningful life for this Iraqi patient? Although we struggle with these same questions with our other Iraqi patients, they are for the most part strangers to us, numbers without voices, who quickly leave our sight and our thoughts. Sabir, with his prolonged stay and development of a persona, has become an emotional liability for his caregivers.

Sabir remains with us and continues to become more of a unique individual, and although he is making progress, his care remains taxing and his future unknown. In this trauma hospital, amidst the chaos of helicopters, operations, and critical care, we keep the wounded alive, both American and Iraqi. But when the chaos clears, reflection inevitably occurs. In caring for patient 4914 and others like him, I have learned that in this war zone medicine for our Iraqi patients is most safely practiced as a myope, well-intentioned but short-sighted, a person who concentrates on the immediate surgery and medication and remains blind to the context of his efforts. While removing pieces of shrapnel, closing bullet holes, and resuscitating those in shock, we can feel content in the knowledge of saving lives but can avoid the unanswerable questions that patients like Sabir make us ask. Sabir, not patient 4914, has forced us to look up from our work, through his dogged presence and force of personality, and acknowledge our frustrations and his uncertain future. As healers, we face the uncomfortable realization that we are asking ourselves, "Are we truly saving you?"

Food for Thought

SUNIL BADVE, MD

In August 1996, I joined Lokmanya Tilak Municipal General Hospital (LTMGH) in Mumbai, India, as an internist–house officer. The LTMGH is well-known for handling medical crises, because it is the largest public hospital in Mumbai Suburban District and is located near Asia's largest slum, Dharavi. Initially, I had a difficult time managing the huge workload. One of the central tasks of the housestaff was to discharge as many patients as possible on preemergency days to make room for the many anticipated admissions on call days. The housestaff who kept their ward census in single digits were most valued. Those who failed to do this invited reproach from the registrars.

One day, the hospital admitted a middle-aged worker with fever, who responded to antimalarial treatment and was soon fit to go home. In the morning of the preemergency day, I filled out his discharge forms and instructed the nurse to discharge him. However, during my evening rounds, I found him still sitting on the hospital bed. He said he was waiting for his ride. I was annoyed, especially because of the anticipated reaction from my registrar. I told the patient that he had been discharged and should leave. I admit I was quite rude to him. The poor man did not argue. I left to attend to other patients, completed my evening rounds, and began to see the new admissions.

Then I witnessed something unforgettable. While the discharged patient sat on his hospital bed, his two small children quietly hid beneath the bed and shared a lip-smacking meal—the hospital food meant for their father. It was obvious from their faces that these children seldom enjoyed such nutritious food. Soon after, the gentleman went home with a satisfied heart and his children with full stomachs.

My heart sank. I was stunned to see that this poor man had overstayed his visit just to feed his children on a day that he could not earn his daily wages because of hospitalization. *Had he done this throughout his hospital stay?* I wondered. That day I learned a lesson not found in *Harrison's Principles of Internal Medicine*—that I was fighting not malaria or any other disease, but the deadliest affliction known to humankind: poverty.

Now, years later, I walk the well-appointed, air-conditioned corridors of P.D. Hinduja National Hospital in Mumbai, India—a privately run, state-of-the-art facility located just three miles from LTMGH. But I am reminded still of poverty—for example, when our kidney transplant recipients stop taking immunosuppression or when patients with end-stage renal disease stop dialysis because of exhausted financial resources. It is a bitter fact that many patients in India prefer to receive inadequate treatment or even stop treatment and die rather than sell their property and burden their family, even when they have a treatable disease.

Now I understand the meaning of the words of wisdom told by my mentor, Dr. Bharat Shah: "What is adequate [treatment] is not practical, so what is practical has to be adequate." As I think back to 1996 and remember the poor man and his two hungry children, I wonder: Do the best practice guidelines and treatment recommendations published in renowned journals really apply to our poor patients?

Medical Ground Zero: An Early Experience of the World Trade Center Disaster

MACK LIPKIN, MD

11 SEPTEMBER 2001

8:50 A.M. Our pregnant chief resident says, "Did you see that the World Trade Center is smoking?"

For years the twin towers of the World Trade Center had guarded Bellevue Hospital's southern horizon.

9:03 A.M. The second tower explodes with flame and smokes heavily, like an upward mudslide. From my wife, "We are okay. I saw the smoke. I'll be in touch."

10:05 A.M. The south tower collapses.

One chief tells me of a senior resident who won't leave her home, distraught because her fiancé works at the World Trade Center and she can't reach him. I call her. Her voice is panicky. She calls back a few minutes later—he ran down 21 flights of stairs, out of the building, and four miles home without stopping. She will come in as soon as she stops shaking.

10:28 A.M. The second tower falls.

This occurs in a distance, without sound or smell.

We truck 5-gallon water cooler bottles with us to 17 West, the medical staging area. Residents mill about. The chief residents organize teams. One resident charges in with news. He has set up a smoke inhalation unit. Another says all admissions should go through the emergency room. Another says patients are being discharged or domiciled in a clinic. The hospital calls an official disaster.

Alumni begin to arrive. Outside volunteers appear. Twenty nursing students in green scrubs flock in. A group of podiatry residents in starchy whites ask what they can do. We send the post-call residents to sleep and set up shifts.

Three senior attendings begin planning, anticipating needs. We review smoke inhalation, carbon monoxide, cyanide, and crush. We assign administrators to phones, to run, and to forage for and guard supplies. Small groups listen to the radio and ponder. Who did this? Who trained them to fly?

Resident experiences flow fast as water. They forget to call home but not to eat. They hoard useful or edible things in their white coats. We order 20 pizzas, cash only: The ATM machines are empty.

The few patients and numerous rescue workers who arrive release puffs of fine gray dust from their clothing. I slip away every 15 minutes to call home. The circuits are busy. An immense emptiness.

1:30 P.M. My beeper goes off.

My wife and daughter are at home with girls from school whose parents couldn't get through. Everyone at home is okay. One father was on the 102nd floor.

We visit each resident team, look them in the eye, and ask how they are doing. We linger longer with those who are trembling. Frantic rumors tell us that we are getting a busload, no, two busloads, but only four patients have been admitted. Post-call residents drift back in to help, unable to sleep.

5:00 P.M. The rescuers can't get in to the victims because the site is too hot.

Barges are going to New Jersey, M.A.S.H units have been set up, but our operating rooms are vacant. Our neurosurgeon rages with his inaction.

An anesthetized, elective surgical patient is woken up to avoid the expected high post-op nursing load. Nonemergent surgeries are canceled, minor operating rooms are converted into major ones, intensive care units are emptied, and 40 homeless patients are discharged to nearby shelters. A Herculean rush to prepare.

Cowboy initiatives begin. Doctors attempt to commandeer transport to go to the site carrying potentially scarce supplies, such as morphine. More volunteers flood in. Probing media eyes seek human-interest stories.

7:00 P.M. The streets are empty except for battalions of rescue vehicles.

The avenues are closed and social boundaries have dissolved. Strangers talk. I go home to little girls with tough questions. Straight answers work best. They stop asking and play.

I need to return to the hospital. The tension between family and serving threatens to break me. The vacated streets flash with emergency lights. I round the eerily empty wards. Through e-mail, 48 friends need to know we are okay, using the Internet to stitch us together. The hospital has seen around 250 persons and has admitted 55—nowhere near enough.

12 SEPTEMBER 2001

Early morning. The hospital's busy—empty duality persists. Some doctors have independently gone to the site or to the M.A.S.H. units. Around the wards, the predominant feeling is of fatigue, futility, and uncertainty. I review trauma literature for noon conference.

Massage therapists offer free massages for staff. The idea tugs a grin of comfort. Everyone needs to help.

Bellevue's entry swarms like an anthill. The morgue expands. Empty refrigerated vans hum. Taped to the entrance wall are 500 missing-persons pictures, posters, and pleas. Journalists, photographers, and TV crews hover like seagulls over broken shells. A tall African faith healer in a kippah massages a grieving woman's aura to her apparent relief. Hundreds line up offering blood.

Competition among helpers is becoming apparent—psychiatry wants to do crisis intervention for our doctors, as does social work and our torture expert. A triage point at the site hears that a fireman with traumatic amputations has been rescued. The emergency medicine docs plan to assess, stabilize, and ambulance him uptown. A fire department medical officer arrives and asserts authority. An intense verbal fight ensues, the fireman arrives, and the fight goes on. He is ambulanced without any basics having been done.

Noon. New York City Emergency Management directs us to stop our entrepreneurs from going to the site. Undisciplined medical people can put themselves and others at risk in the rubble, they claim. Those who do go cite unmet needs, especially at night. A surgical team extracted a pinned rescue worker and saved his legs. The Bellevue medical director prohibits further teams from going.

Three site triage points spring up. Team members wash eyes, patch abrasions and burns, and give nebulizer treatments. Our cardiac care unit director, a single mother, joins the team at Engine 10. Her father had served there, and she knows several of the firemen. Her fireman brother has not been heard from. She will return there for five days, finding her brother alive on day 3.

Ward teams arrange support discussions. One deeply anxious resident's significant other has gone down to the site and hasn't been in touch. She can't concentrate, cries, and hasn't slept.

Fire marshals assigned to the morgue to identify firemen sit for hours in a lower purgatory of smoke and burned flesh—12 hours on, 12 hours off.

Leaving the hospital means passing long lines of missing-person seekers. An NBC News truck is covered with photographs of the missing. Smoke is in the air.

We each need to help, and the helpers are competing.

13 SEPTEMBER 2001

Residents in a support group begin their discussion. "Out there is so strange." "The missing-persons wall broke me up." "I take 2 hours to write a progress note." "Normal things startle me." "I have no patience for trivia." "I felt better going home even though there were paw prints in the ashes." Sounds normally unheard evoke fear and vigilance.

We try to revert to a normal schedule. Clinics reopen but are empty.

An internist goes to Ground Zero, for himself. Darkness alternating with brilliant lights obscures the devastating visual impact, cocooning the workers. He joins a band of doctors wandering around offering services to rescue workers, glad to improvise small acts of healing.

As I go home, a homeless man lectures on the advantages of the street. A rescue worker sleeps soundly over a vent, looking homeless.

Judgment takes a hind seat to needs for usefulness and impulse. Everyone salves uncertainty with action and information. The absence of patients is a dark hole we attempt to fill. Brittle, we feel the infinite yet individual aftershocks.

14 SEPTEMBER 2001

Picture IDs are enforced at the hospital, and visitors are turned away. Patients without appointment slips are hassled. A bomb scare at the medical examiner's office results in an evacuation of medical school buildings. The top deans forget to call the bottom ones, who forget to call the students. Events spawn theories and hierarchies. Who considers whom expendable stains goodwill and renews social boundaries. Bellevue feels slighted by the barging of victims to New Jersey. The New York University Hospital envies Bellevue's place as medical epicenter. Futility enough for all.

At a medical housestaff conference, everyone shares experiences of loss of concentration, repetition, avoidance, startle, sadness, and intrusive anger. Meetings metastasize.

The New York University Downtown Hospital has seen almost 1000 persons, has been running on emergency generators, and may close or transfer patients. We gear up again, putting all residents on call for the weekend. Some residents, especially those with spouses or families, feel ashamed that they resent sentry duty against the absent onslaught.

Talking heads on television pale beside intense reality.

17 SEPTEMBER 2001

The missing-persons wall has become a shrine with candles, flowers, and pictures over pictures that scream desperation and hope. I watch refreshed staff stiffen as they see the wall.

In the wards, openness, leadership flexibility, and goodwill are dissolving. There is an almost rigid desire to be back to things as usual.

18 SEPTEMBER 2001

A staff member's daughter seeks counseling. She lives alone near the site. She begins and ends each symptom with "I don't know if this is normal or not." It all seems normal. I listen mostly, ask for more, respond empathically to her suffering, and explain, once I think I have heard it fully, that each of her symptoms makes sense in the setting of this threat, that she is re-establishing her world.

20 SEPTEMBER 2001

Nightmares begin for many.

Our medical students are active. They compile the city's first list of post-attack hospital admissions. They go to the site to wash eyes, hand out food, help transporters. At the medical examiner's office, they talk with those missing someone, scribe, set up systems, help take dental x-rays, sort body parts, take DNA specimens, and plan a memorial service.

Another meeting with Bellevue attendings. A dedicated, selfless HIV *maven* is angry that her AIDS patients request Viagra, survivor biology resurging chemically. Another attending has volunteered to work with families missing someone. Her father was an architect of the World Trade Center. His nostalgia grieves his daughter.

21 SEPTEMBER 2001

How will we counsel persons who are afraid of what may come next when we are also afraid? We are still preparing for a marathon and for coming events; we need to take care of ourselves to remain strong and available; and if dealing with trauma is traumatic, there is help available. My own black hole of uncertainty widens.

We receive a request to provide medical backup for the family assistance and counseling center on Pier 94. The grief counselors want primary care physicians available for medical complications they fear may arise. We brace ourselves for a new trauma: the issuance of death certificates without bodies.

The pier, with its "one-stop shopping for all victims' needs," is overwhelming. Two newly carpeted acres, hundreds of cubicles, every imaginable agency. Remarkably New York—teeming, energetic, busy, tightly organized, fresh flowers on every desk and counter, and good food for victims and staff. It is friendly for families and set up well for all varieties of counseling. We sit with Red Cross nurses from San Diego, Houston, and Tokyo. We see normal primary care problems, neglected chronic disease, and startlingly diverse hypochondriasis. A special police unit that trains a bald eagle walks around, the therapy dogs spooking the eagle.

My daughter and I go to the playground. Three police cars rush by going uptown with full sirens. My daughter pauses her rope jumping and asks, "Is something else falling down?"

22 SEPTEMBER 2001

Still, the world is real and intensely beautiful. We hug a lot. My daughter has been building little houses all over the place. "New York lost its two front teeth," she says, her grin showing two gaps where canines came out three weeks ago, "but they will grow back."

On Becoming
A Doctor

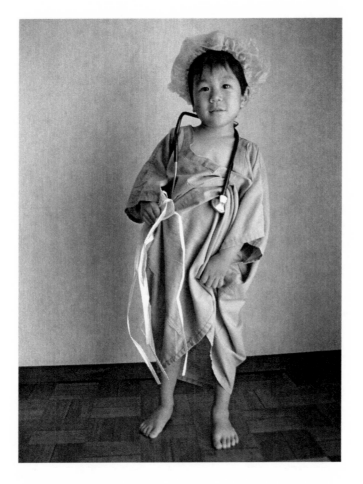

Learning Medicine Through the Closet Door

J. RANDALL CURTIS, MD, MPH

The year was 1986. I was on my first rotation as a third-year medical student. It was 7 P.M. on my first night on-call. I had picked up my patient for the night: a 35-year-old woman with a long history of type 1 diabetes who had suffered many of the ravages of that disease. As I leaned over *Harrison's Principles of Internal Medicine* in the team room trying to figure out what else to write in my admission note, the intern received a call about an admission coming from an outside hospital. The patient was a 42-year-old gay man who presented to a community hospital with a headache and stiff neck. A spinal tap revealed fungal meningitis, which, at that time, was very unusual. The community hospital was transferring the patient to the university hospital where I was in training.

When the intern got off the phone, he turned to the two other medical students on our team to fill them in. All three of his medical students were male, so the intern felt free to use graphic and derogatory language to describe the patient, his sexual orientation, and the sexual activities that would most likely have led to his HIV infection. I sat in the corner of the room with my eyes fixed on my textbook, feeling my face grow warm, staring at the blur of black and white on the page, but unable to read a word, for what seemed like ages.

Throughout the evening, the patient was referred to simply as "the fag." Both of my classmates were waiting for their admission for the night, but neither wanted to take care of this particular patient.

I was presumed heterosexual, not by default, but because I actually told my classmates that I was heterosexual. I had moved thousand of miles to go to one of the best and, in some ways, most conservative medical schools in the country. I wanted to fit in. I wanted to be judged for my abilities, not my sexual orientation. I didn't think that my sexual orientation was anyone's business except my own. But I also wanted recognition for my 12-year relationship with my partner. I considered my long-term relationship as more defining of who I was than the fact that my partner, like myself, was a man. So I told my classmates that I was married to a woman. I even gave them my partner's real name, since it was a name used by men and women.

The first call night of my third year of medical school wasn't the first time that I felt intensely uncomfortable because of homophobic comments, but it was the most memorable for two reasons: the intern's anger about his new patient and my experience the following morning.

On rounds the next morning, as our team was outside the door of the gay man with meningitis, I listened intently to his presentation, physical findings, and lab results. I was developing a keen interest in HIV medicine because I identified with these men. I hadn't yet had a close friend develop AIDS, but I felt drawn to understand this disease.

I followed behind my team as we entered the room. When I looked at the man in the bed, I found myself looking at a friend. I had met Peter at the Gay and Lesbian Community Center. Six months earlier, I had been to Thanksgiving dinner at the home of Peter and his partner, James. In the same instant that I recognized Peter, I found myself backing out of the room and into the hall. I stood with my back against the wall and listened to the pounding of my heart. When my team came out of the room, I resumed morning rounds without a word to anyone. To this day, I am surprised that, at that moment, I was more concerned about myself than about Peter.

Later that morning, I went back to see Peter. He had seen me back out of his room. He asked me if I were "out" at medical school, but I believe he knew the answer before I spoke. That was all that was said about my reaction that morning. I sat on his bed and asked him how he was feeling and what I could do to help. I felt as if Peter were taking care of me, rather than me taking care of him. He told me that the intern said he would need a repeat spinal tap and asked me if I would do it. I was taken abeck by the request but surprised myself by quickly assenting. I never discussed the intern's comments with Peter, but Peter instinctively knew that he did not want that intern to provide any of his care. I agreed.

In the following days, I performed the spinal tap, drew blood, and put in IVs. I spent a lot of time in his room explaining the diagnostic tests and treatment recommendations. I never did sit quietly holding his hand. I never did share with Peter my feelings about his illness or seeing him in the hospital bed on that first morning.

Peter went home after seven days. I visited him a half-dozen times before he died. I remember him walking around the house with his IV pole, calling it his "dancing partner". He used to say he liked his IV pole because it didn't run over his toes as often as James did when they danced together. He didn't come back to the university hospital, although he was hospitalized twice more before he died. I never found the time to visit him when he was in the community hospital.

More than ten years have gone by since I walked in on morning rounds to discover Peter in that hospital bed. Several months ago, I found myself sitting on a screened porch in Nova Scotia in the pouring rain, telling a circle of new friends how I had become interested in trying to improve the quality of care for patients dying of AIDS. As I told the story of Peter's first hospitalization, I suddenly realized that Peter had asked me to care for him in the only way that I was capable of: by putting in his IVs, doing his spinal tap, and drawing his blood. I wasn't capable, at that time, of caring in the way that I really wanted to: sitting on the edge of his bed, holding his hand, and being with him. I see that as one of the consequences of learning medicine through the closet door.

A Palindrome

PAULA TATARUNIS, MD

Ignaz Semmelweis,
who cut the maternal death rate
in the *Allgemeines Krankenhaus*
obstetrical ward
from 18 to 1.2 percent
by insisting that the doctors
wash their hands
before and after
each exam and delivery,
so outraged his colleagues
by his findings
that they hounded him
back to Budapest
where he wrote
Die Aetiology der Begriff
und die Prophylaxis des Kindbedfiebers
and, in 1865, died of sepsis
in an insane asylum,
a brokenman.

In Brockelman's Market,
a women, pregnant,
her blouse a color
between faded yellow
and yellowed white,
between spit-up milk
and rebleached diapers,
a tired woman, who, soon,
for the sixth time, won't
die of childbed fever,
is buying warm
whiterolls.

A Rose for Dr. Martin

MICHAEL J. SCHOTT, MA, MLS

I am the clinical medical librarian at a teaching hospital, who sits in the back during morning report while medical residents tell their tales to the attending physician. It is a time when teacher–physicians fill white boards with chief complaints, physical exams, lab values, and drug regimens and try to coax correct answers out of sleep-deprived residents.

I have sat in the back of the room at morning report for over 15 years at two different hospitals in two states. My job is to listen to the stories, record the facts to find the supporting literature, talk to residents, and fix an occasional ailing PDA. Mostly, I sit in the back and listen with the pharmacy residents, a silent audience to the life-and-death drama that unfolds every day in teaching hospitals all over the world. Moved by many of the stories, I can do nothing but sit and listen, fascinated by the craft of the healing arts.

One doctor knows my heart. Shelda Martin read an article I wrote called "Notes from Morning Report: On the Bleeding Edge of Medicine." Her empathy for my station is obvious in her dealings with me. She is very patient. During a lecture I gave on using PDAs that she attended, I made a comment about being passed EKG strips in morning report but being unable to understand them. I would peer at the strips like an archeologist examining ancient runes, trying to understand their hidden meaning. I have tried to understand those strips that somehow tell the secrets of patients' hearts, but with little success. Books on the topic, written for scientists and not librarians, have been little help.

One day after my PDA lecture, at the end of the morning report, when the residents had scattered to attend to their patients or catch a little sleep, Dr. Martin approached me. She said, "I'm going to teach you how to read an EKG." I was shocked that she would take time out of her busy day to teach me. It seemed almost sacrilegious to me, like a master magician sharing her art with a member of the audience. I tried to shy away, afraid to reveal my ignorance. She started with EKG lead placement and spent 20 minutes explaining to me what an EKG does. She showed me how the heart works and how the electrical impulses from the heart travel. She showed me the P wave, the QRS complex, and the spaces between the beats. She was patient. She answered every question. She listened.

In the process of touching her heart to make a point, she touched mine. Suddenly it made sense to me. Struck by the kindness this gracious physician showed, I was fertile ground for her detailed explanations. I started to understand. Having seen the worst of medicine on more than one occasion, it is easy to recognize the best.

In 15 years, no other physician had ever taken the time to do that for me. It was a random act of kindness that this librarian will always remember. Thank you, Dr. Martin. In the end, you need no rose. Your fine colors are made brilliant by your actions. You are a rose of your profession.

Joan's Education

MARYANN OVERLAND, BA

There was a wad of bubblegum stuck to the upper right corner of
Joan's windshield. From the looks of it, the gum had seen better days.
Baked-on greasy streaks ran from the pink blob to the dashboard and
told of countless seasons of climatic abuse. Every morning as she
climbed into her 1993 Volvo, Naugahyde seat cracking and groaning
under her increasing weight, Joan cursed her ex-boyfriend and made a
mental note to clean the gum off the glass when she got home. As she
buckled her seat belt, she noticed the roll of fat creeping over her for-
merly slim waistline and made the second, soon-to-be-broken promise
of the young day: to get some exercise. But time passed and the wad of
gum, like any good piece of performance art, continued to evolve.
Joan viewed it as a daily reminder of her shortcomings. Her body
became softer, doughier, and the lines around her eyes only hinted at
the degree of her weariness.

Joan did not think it inappropriate that she had missed her grandfather's funeral for fear of skipping a week of anatomy labs. Nor did
she worry when she declined an entire summer of her closest friends'
weddings, or note that her first nephew was nearly walking before she
met him. Seldom did her mind wander to when—or if—she might fit
in a romance of her own. Joan no longer returned personal phone calls

or e-mails. She didn't allow herself to count the number of months that had passed since her last real conversation with her best friend. She did not stop to consider that she just might not have a best friend anymore. She understood that a career in medicine meant making sacrifices. Her mind was occupied with pharmacology and physiology, biosynthetic pathways and differential diagnoses. Oh, occasionally, as she was drifting off to much-needed sleep, her thoughts would dreamily turn to a different life: hiking with friends in Yosemite, learning to surf in Bolinas, backpacking through Spain, driving cross country with the windows down, the stereo blasting, and the wind in her hair. Her semi-conscious mind would take her to times of late-night concerts and the intoxication of new love. But in the morning when the alarm startled her out of sleep at an ungodly hour, all memory of her past life receded back to her Rolodex of forgotten joy.

It was a bone-chilling Wednesday in February when Joan met Alicia, an angry yet hauntingly beautiful 16-year-old girl, at the pediatrician's office where she was doing a rotation. Alicia had fainted twice in school that week, and her mom had dragged her into the office to find out what was wrong. As Joan walked toward the exam room, she rapidly ran through the differential for syncope. There could be a cardiac etiology—bradyarrhythmia or tachyarrhythmia, a neurologic or psychogenic disorder, orthostatic hypotension, hypoglycemia, hypoxemia, a seizure disorder, hypocalcemic or alkalotic tetany, hyperventilation. She also reminded herself to inquire privately about whether Alicia might be pregnant.

As she entered the room, Joan saw a too-thin girl stretched out on the exam table with fuchsia hair peeking out from under the hood of an oversized sweatshirt. Alicia lay with her arms across her face, as though the glow from the flat fluorescent light was simply too much to bear. A fleeting reflection passed through Joan's mind: "I used to be that girl." She quickly regained her poise and proceeded with the visit. After talking for a few minutes with Alicia and her mother, Joan asked the mother to give them some privacy.

She took Alicia's blood pressure on her right arm. She asked about Alicia's eating habits, whether she was sexually active, her last menstrual period, how often she was exercising, and whether she had any accompanying symptoms or warning signs before she fainted. The teen answered this string of queries with flat "yeahs" and "nopes," all the while avoiding eye contact. Joan did not notice. She did a quick yet thorough head, eyes, ears, nose, and throat exam. Joan maintained a calculated emotional distance from the patient. She struggled not to reveal her growing frustration at her inability to unlock the secret of this problem. Tail between her legs, Joan started to leave the room to consult with the attending physician. She felt like she was missing something, and if she could only ask the right question or perform the appropriate exam, the diagnosis would be obvious.

As she began to turn the handle on the door, she was flooded with a wave of emotion, of empathy, of memory. She flashed back to being 16 years old, alone, angry at the world and unable to cope. She recalled feeling like adults couldn't begin to grasp the depth of the despair, and guiltily dredged up the pledge she had made never to forget what it was like to be 16 and suffering.

She turned and fixed her eyes on Alicia, sitting on the exam table, staring at her scuffed-up, black Chuck Taylors. "I wonder what she's thinking about right now," Joan wondered. "Does she know how scared I am? Scared that I won't be able to figure this out, scared that I'm not any good at this?" She began to speak.

"Alicia ...."

She looked at the sullen teen, who was now defiantly glaring at her with obvious mistrust and disappointment. Joan sat down on the stool and began again.

"Alicia, what's wrong?"

There was a long pause. Joan was uncomfortable with the silence, but she forced herself to endure it. She counted to 5. Then 10. Then 20. Alicia, eyes now narrowed to slits, finally opened her mouth to speak.

"I dunno. You're the medical student. You figure it out."

Joan tried again. "I don't mean with the fainting. I mean in general. What's wrong? What's going on in your life that's making you so unhappy?" Joan put down the chart and pen, unwrapped the nooselike stethoscope from around her neck, shrugged off her white coat, and said, "Tell me."

Alicia considered the question and opened her mouth as if to speak, but then closed it again. The silence was almost unbearable. "Go ahead, you can tell me," Joan repeated. Again Alicia opened her mouth and shut it quickly. Finally words began to spill out. Words about the pressure to be thin and beautiful and perfect. About feeling inconsequential and powerless. About frustration with the world. About injustice. About loneliness, confusion, anguish. She talked about forced sex and shame. She told of not being able to eat, sleep, or connect with other people. She told about the gulf between herself and her family. In a few brief moments, the girl's words reminded Joan why she had left her previous career to go into medicine.

Joan didn't realize she was crying until the salty taste in her mouth was too strong to ignore. She was crying for Alicia, but even more, she was crying for herself. Crying for the distance she had strayed from her vision of what it meant to be a healer, and crying because she hadn't realized it until now. She resisted the voice in her head that told her she was being unprofessional, and allowed herself to weep with Alicia until they were both out of tears.

On her drive home, Joan turned off National Public Radio and popped in a Pavement CD. It had been months since she had taken a vacation from "All Things Considered." "Just for today I don't need to know," she mused. When she got home, she walked in the house, picked up the Goo-Be-Gone and a razor blade, returned to the Volvo, and finally removed that goddamn wad of gum from her windshield.

Trouble

BEATRIZ M. RODRIGUEZ, MD

The trouble with Med students is
they are young,
not young like spring time
but young like a morning,
full of possibility
full of questions you have stopped asking.
And sometimes they look at you with this
admiration that seems misdirected.
They are lean, they haven't yet inhaled the
stale donuts and coffee of the 3 a.m. ICU.
They are still reverent about death and admire
your irreverence.
The trouble with Med students is they follow
you around, they page you, they work to keep
up with you,
you work to stay ahead.
The trouble is they stop you, they look in your eyes
and they ask.
The trouble with Med students is they touch you

and make you feel something.
And that is a bittersweet thing, for we haven't time to
feel, but to feel is such a sweet memory that it is in a
way quite exhilarating and you find you have wasted time
with it.
Then at night when exhausted ... you lie ... you remember that
feeling and wonder where it came from and if it will come
again.
And in the early morning madness of rounds you look, perhaps too
        expectantly,
for that young face of morning.
And you check yourself and self-admonish.
But still you look for that face.
And recall that strange look your own teachers used to
give you, part awe, part irritation
and you smile at the legacy.

Of Poems and Patients

DAVID SEDER, MD

I was thinking tonight about how we move through a lot of worlds in a short time. My wife and I were out listening to a folk singer, and I realized how hard it is to listen to live music without leaning across a bar. It wasn't so long ago that four or five nights a week I poured beer and shook drinks while customers came and went, and not so long since I knew hundreds of people across a tall oak bar by face, voice, or drink of choice. That life is so different from my current one that it could have been led by another person entirely.

I was a pretty good bartender. Not masterful with drinks but good with space, ambiance, and friendliness, at making regulars feel at home and at taking care of them. I worked the same bar for six years and, at intervals, filched from it, fixed it, loved it, ran it, and finally just worked the shows as a means of paying for college and a new baby. For years afterward, I never went into a bar because it was all too familiar to enjoy. I began my "career" as a poet, then played at boxing and business, and at age 27 left the bar world for good by going to medical school.

Last month, in my new role as a doctor, I helped to kill a patient. I've not been blamed, and she was desperately ill, but I can still see the bright arterial blood pumping out of her chest from an artery I tore. With no platelets to close the tear, she bled and bled, through twelve units of blood. Finally, at 3 o'clock in the morning, a chest surgeon cauterized the artery in the OR, and she came back to the ICU sicker, although it's hard to believe, than when I had first been called to her bedside nine hours earlier. She died four days later; her death certificate did not mention my misadventure. There are a lot of things I would change about this case, but the time to do so is gone. Although a dozen or more people were involved, probably only I still care about the injury I caused, and I don't particularly want to let it go.

The folk singer at the bar had a beautiful voice that wrapped around you, and I thought about being up on a stage reading poetry, about some beauty that I myself had created years ago. A long time has passed since then, and I don't know if I still create beauty through my work or not. It was a conscious decision to walk away from the arts and go into medicine. I wanted a job with tangible, practical results. Now I can often get a patient's pulse back, move quickly through the paces of resuscitation, unravel a tricky diagnosis. Sometimes, I help people cope with grief or I get a student excited about medicine. I like to think that I help more people than I harm. Yet, as I listened to the singer's liquid voice, it seemed like giving up poetry for medicine was a poor trade.

As a bartender, at times I had to deal with troublemakers, and I did not shy away from fistfighting. It was necessary to protect the customers, and I only used violence as a last resort. Sometimes things were clear-cut but, as in medicine, not always. At times I experienced the dull nausea of regret from things that hadn't gone as well as I had hoped, or from the feeling that perhaps I had in some way contributed to the problem I was "solving." The practice afterward was the same: to stand up and take responsibility, to hold myself accountable, to explain the motivations, the reasons, and the actions one step at a time. None of us is perfect, but we can all be held to a certain standard of competence and behavior.

I don't miss bartending, but if I left medicine, I would mourn its loss as I've mourned the passage of my poetry. On a daily basis, it is both a privilege and a joy to have the trust of patients and their families and the camaraderie of peers. There is no challenge to make your blood race like that of a difficult case, no mind game as rigorous as the challenging differential diagnosis, and though the stakes are high, so are the rewards. Still, a fine poem has a purity that this trade will never match and creates moments of lightness that I have not felt now in years. I don't ever, as a poet, remember having held a life in my hands and watched it fall through my fingers and crack upon the floor. I will never get used to this, and I will not let it go, because I don't think life can matter unless death matters.

As a doctor, I want very much for life to matter.

Present Tense

STAN SCHUMAN, MD, DrPH

At lecture's end,
The graying professor sees
150 medical students
Charge the exit for lunch.
Gathering slides, he wonders
If his 50 minutes worked.
How to link biochemistry
To preventive medicine?
Could these bright novices
Follow the essential logic?
Relating amino acids
To protein layers of the eye,
To optics of cornea and lens,
To cataract formation in sunlight,
Disabling peasants in India
Where one needs enough sight
To hoe and harvest, or else
The family starves, in one season,
Unless someone cares, and
Does lens repair.

Why expect exam-driven students
To follow such reasoning, or want to?
Why ask a freshman to see himself
As a full-fledged surgeon,
Cool and competent,
Preventing blindness-and-hunger
Among rice-field families overseas?
How unlikely, the teacher admits,
That 50 minutes could hint
Such a future.

Pondering the limits of learning,
The professor thinks of Eric,
Longtime friend, master-carpenter,
And how he may feel, at day's end.
Leaning against his pickup in the driveway
Of a two-story nearly complete,
Glancing over his shoulder,
Into the setting sun,
At trim soffits and roofline,
Proof of his expertise,
Hardly noting his pony-tailed apprentice,
Tan and lean, lighting into his jeep,
Tearing into a sixpack,
Maxing the stereo, and
Blasting down the highway ...

The highway of youth, where
Carpenters- and doctors-to-be,
Occupy the present tense,
First person.

Thoughts from Gross Anatomy

ERIC MICHAEL DAVID, JD

The day she visited the dissecting room
They had four men laid out, black as burnt turkey,
Already half unstrung. A vinegary fume
Of the death vats clung to them [...]
And she could scarcely make out anything
In that rubble of skull plates and old leather.
A sallow piece of string held it together.

Sylvia Plath, *Two Views of a Cadaver Room*

The words sat so unremarkably on the page: "The cadaver should be transected between T12 and L1." Straightforward. Direct—like directions for heating a frozen dinner. I had been quite pressed for time that day, as anyone who recalls their first year of medical school will probably appreciate, so I had not read the dissection procedures before coming to lab. I could not believe that such a remarkable event would be presented so unassumingly. I turned to one of my anatomy partners and, pointing to the passage on the rather stained, well-worn page, inquired, "You don't think they actually mean ..."

She nodded gravely. "Yes. Cut her in half."

We had been dissecting for almost 8 weeks, having completed our exploration of the thorax and abdomen, and we had all grown quite comfortable with the experience of dissecting a fellow human being. Growing up with a grandfather, father, and four uncles who are physicians, a course in Human Anatomy was an experience I somehow always knew I would have—an experience I welcomed. "There's always some clown who just has to play jump-rope with a length of small bowel," my father had warned me. But in our two months of dissection, I had never seen my classmates exhibit anything but great respect for their cadavers. Indeed, how grateful we all were to these people for granting us such a profound gift, enabling an educational opportunity that would last us our entire careers. Yet as I looked about the lab at my classmates removing their saws and chisels from the drawers beneath the dissection tables, I felt that the entire dynamic of our first-year experience was about to change.

A classmate of mine approached from a table on the other side of the lab. She was visibly troubled. Putting her hand on my shoulder, she whispered, "Eric, I *cannot* do this. Think," she demanded, "think of the *sound* it's going to make." I did. I knew exactly what it would sound like: dissonance in the purest sense. I left the anatomy lab. I needed a moment alone to consider what I was about to do.

"Have you named her yet? Did you name your cadaver?" a friend had asked weeks earlier, after my first day of medical school. I had not anticipated how very curious all of my "civilian" friends would be about my anatomy course.

"Well, no," I replied, "I mean, I'm reasonably sure she already had a name, and it seems disrespectful to give her another."

"What was it like the first time you cut into her flesh?" another friend inquired.

"Disarming," I answered, reflecting on how much tougher the skin was than I had anticipated, how much work was required to make that first cut.

"Did you ... did you actually hold her heart in your hands?" my 9-year-old cousin asked tentatively. "Because that just seems ... wrong."

For eight weeks, dinner and phone conversations with all my "civilian" friends inevitably turned to anatomy. I often tried to change the subject, only to find myself confronted by "just how long is the small intestine?" or "what does cancer look like?" Anytime I met someone and told them I was a first-year medical student, their immediate response was, "What's Anatomy like?" Yet despite everyone's intense curiosity, I was amazed to see subtle changes in relationships with people I had known my whole life. My "civilian" friends and relatives began to treat me as someone who had seen something he was not supposed to see, something that was fundamentally forbidden.

Irving Stone, writing about Michelangelo's experiences in dissecting cadavers, offered that, in performing the act, the artist was inherently changed with respect to his peers—transformed by "the happiness that arises out of knowledge, for now he knew about the most vital organ of the body, what it looked like, how it felt." A friend of mine summed it up quite eloquently: "You know what the difference is between doctors and everyone else? Doctors have seen what's on the other side of the bellybutton. So many of us spend our whole lives looking down at our bellybutton and thinking, What the heck is back there? Does it lead into my stomach? Is it connected to some sort of tube? Is there a tiny little knot tied in the back? We don't know! But you've seen what's back there. To have that demystified fundamentally changes you with respect to everyone else."

As I prepared myself to return to the anatomy lab, I contemplated whether sawing another human being in half was a more profound demystification than I desired. Before starting medical school, I directed a documentary about the Cold War. During a tour of a government facility, I quite inadvertently wandered into a room filled with about a dozen nuclear warheads in various stages of disassembly. As I reentered the anatomy lab that day and was confronted with 30 transected bodies, I was so vividly reminded of that room filled with "transected" nuclear warheads. As striking and incongruous as the analogy may seem, it was the only other time I had been directly confronted by entities once so powerful, so significant, so functional, now rendered so profoundly impotent.

The act of human dissection may very well be the one event that distinguishes physicians from nonphysicians in a very real way. It is an experience that is remembered with varying degrees of fondness, and with emotions ranging from fascination to disgust. Indeed, the entire process is intensified by the trepidation we students experience in examining and then utterly dismantling our very first patient. Dissection of a fellow human being is not simply the solution to the great mystery of what lies behind the bellybutton, but it is an act so taboo that it is criminalized outside the medical context. There are some things in medicine for which one can never prepare—things to which one can never fundamentally grow accustomed: the birth of an anencephalic infant, overseeing the autopsy of a patient with whom one had been conversing only hours previously, and, perhaps, cutting a fellow human being in half. As I grasped the saw that day, I pondered what a strange and wondrous profession I was about to enter.

Past and Present

KEITH WRENN, MD

I went to a meeting this week and confronted my past. I went to see if I could learn anything new about electrocardiograms. The room was full of internists of all ages. Most were there for a final cramming session before they took a test that would supposedly pronounce them competent at reading tracings, or not. This test, it seems, would ensure their continued ability to bill for electrocardiogram interpretation.

Several smart young cardiologists filled the hours with a mix of fact and impression. With computerized slide presentations and laser pointers, they talked about how an ST segment's appearance indicated ischemia or injury and whether the ST segment was nonspecific. They listed the criteria for hypertrophy of each chamber and for distinguishing between supraventricular tachycardia with aberration and ventricular tachycardia. They told us how to tell pericarditis from early repolarization and how to tell artifact from reality. They were smart, efficient, and often funny. And I learned some things.

As luck would have it, the long-retired, former chairman of medicine at the institution where I trained was scheduled to speak at the end of the course. While I gathered a Danish and coffee in the interval before he spoke, I approached him. He smiled warmly, recognized me, and asked about my partner, who had also trained with him. He seemed genuinely pleased that I had made the effort. It was clear that his 80-plus years had taken their toll. I had heard he had new knees. He didn't seem as tall as I remembered, and he was very hard of hearing despite hearing aids.

Before he began his talk, he stumbled slightly, trying to maneuver the overhead projector into place, and he had trouble getting the laser pointer to work. The room was quiet and cold.

Then he looked up and started to speak. His voice was deep, but quiet, with a measured southern lilt. It commanded attention and not a little fear. He had large hands that he used sparingly but effectively. He glanced at the electrocardiogram on the screen, and you could almost see his eyes spark. I was suddenly transported back 25 years to a large conference room filled with white-coated interns and residents like myself.

He was from a different time, when the physical examination actually meant something. When almost everything you needed came from the bedside, and you didn't always need an echocardiogram or a scan. He drew the QRS, T, and ST segment vectors on an overhead projector. He spoke of shifting axis and ruptured plaque; of the "fan," not "bundle," of conducting tissue in the left ventricle; of the course of each of the major coronary arteries; of how he would correlate the electrocardiogram changes with the anatomic changes, either from catheterization, autopsy, or the knowing production of septal infarcts in hypertrophic cardiomyopathy. And he predicted very specifically where the particular coronary artery had finally failed in its duty ... "around the junction of the first and middle thirds of the left anterior descending artery."

Often he would call residents up to the front of the room and have us draw the vectors. After our usually flawed attempts, he would lower his head and shake it sadly. "How can this be?" he'd say and sigh as he corrected our drawings.

As the next electrocardiogram went up on the screen, a doctor next to me snorted derisively, snapping me back to the present. "There he goes again with those vectors," she said with a roll of her eyes. I sensed she thought that his talk was irrelevant, perhaps quaint. We used to joke about him too, probably for similar reasons. We just couldn't keep up with him. The difference was in the respect he commanded at the time.

I went to a meeting this week and confronted my past. I saw a mentor from long ago who demanded excellence from his students and residents, as well as himself. Who never took shortcuts and who didn't speak primarily in sound bites. Who had immersed himself in the science of medicine. Over his entire career he had done the long hours of dissection and correlation and thinking. He continued to learn and write long after most of us will be alive, let alone practicing. And despite, or maybe because of, his years, he was still, by far, the smartest person in the room. A few may think medicine has passed him by, but I say it just never caught up with him.

That Intern Dream

JACK COULEHAN, MD

I had the intern dream again last night,
restored to white, but decades older
than that group of docs I hadn't met.

Halfway through, it seemed I kept
clutching a fear so tight, my smile was tin.
Nor had I seen a single patient yet.

At midnight rumpled interns ate
cold spaghetti, bread and juice. From a seat
across the room, I scanned their faces,

convinced they didn't know my hideous sin.
In fact, I had never learned to put
a tube in place, or make an incision.

Instead I read a book. Emergency!
My name was called. A code. I had to run,
but which direction? The route I took

was wrong, and I reversed. My pants collapsed.
My coat and shirt were gone. I jockeyed
to the corridor in underpants and socks.

What chance I had of saving face was lost.
The call was cardiac. My father lay
gasping for his breath, but I'd never seen

a Swan put in, or learned resuscitation.
Emptiness arose. I ran away.
Lilies choked the room. I slept. I woke.

A Lesson from the Third Year

ERIC HELMS, MD

During my medicine clerkship, I had the privilege of caring for a man whose case brought up many questions and dilemmas in my mind. Mr. L. was a 70-year-old Chinese man who spoke only Cantonese, and in a dialect that most translators found incomprehensible. He apparently had no family and was in this country illegally. He lived with a group of other Chinese people, all of whom worked for a restaurant and lived with the owners. It was questionable whether Mr. L. had ever seen a western doctor before. He presented to the emergency department with severe abdominal pain, having not voided in some time.

The doctors determined that Mr. L. had a urinary obstruction secondary to benign prostatic hypertrophy. They relieved this problem through catheterization, but Mr. L.'s kidneys functioned so poorly that the doctors thought Mr. L. had some form of chronic renal failure as well. A doctor performed a renal biopsy that showed severe glomerulosclerosis, and renal failure was imminent. Dialysis was begun promptly. After learning of his condition, the owners of the restaurant declined to assume care for the man. They refused to allow him to continue residing with the other workers or to provide transportation. Since no other family or friends could be found to provide care, Mr. L. sat in the hospital for weeks and then months awaiting an indefinite placement to a nursing facility that would arrange for his dialysis.

I joined in this story several days after the patient's initial admission. The case was confusing, not so much from a medical standpoint but from the perspective of preserving the patient's dignity and quality of life.

The most obvious barriers to care in this case were language and culture. The hospital had 24-hour access to a telephone translator, but I realized quickly that this service was not being used. It seemed like most of the doctors and nurses were either ignoring Mr. L., perhaps uncomfortable with the language barrier, or doing quick exams in which the subjective response was inferred. The typical progress note for Mr. L. was something along the lines of "Patient Chinese speaking. No c/o ... ." Interestingly, Mr. L. was receiving no medicine for pain. A physician had written an order for as-needed pain medicine, but Mr. L. couldn't communicate his pain. I found no indication that anyone had made the effort to ask. When I dialed up the translator on my first day, Mr. L. reported that he was extremely uncomfortable.

Second, I realized that even with translation, Mr. L.'s comprehension and insight were extremely poor. I spent many hours explaining things and obtaining consents. Mr. L. never had any questions. When I stopped to ask, "Do you understand? Do you have questions? What do you think of this?" Mr. L. always gave one response to the translator. "If Doctor thinks this is best ... ." Eventually, it dawned on me that Mr. L. just wasn't getting it. Either he was in denial, or he never really understood. As the picture became more dire, he began asking me questions without any sense of irony: "How many more times must I go to dialysis?" "When can I go back to live with my friends?" and "Will I leave today?" My heart broke as I realized I would have to be the one to disappoint him.

Throughout the whole ordeal, I think Mr. L.'s biggest complaint was about his Foley catheter. He *hated* it and could never understand why he needed it. At one point, he tried to pull it out. I don't think Mr. L. ever knew what a prostate, kidneys, or a nursing home were.

Finally, I saw Mr. L.'s ultimate disposition as a tragedy that I continue to question. At the time, no one seemed comfortable addressing my questions about the patient's placement and the possibility of a transplant. The reactions I got ranged from shared concern to indifference to anger. *Don't you understand that the hospital is eating all the cost for this guy? He's lucky we don't put him on a plane back to China.* This was what some seemed to imply.

What a sad and lonely outcome: to be relegated to a state nursing facility where he could speak to no one and had limited understanding of the reason for his placement. I could picture it as a prison of both the mind and the body—and in our zeal to be doctors, we handed Mr. L. that sentence.

What was our responsibility to this man who lived in this country illegally and had no ability to pay? Should he be eligible for a transplant? Should we blame the other workers and the restaurant owner for not taking him back? They had used his labor while he was healthy, but turned their backs on him when he became sick. Was all of this "care" even what the patient desired? If he truly understood the implications for his future life, perhaps he would not have always assented to the "Doctor."

My role in this story was to offer the only things I had as a student—my time, my ear, and my voice. I took time every day to use the translator to ask Mr. L. how he was, to tell him what to expect, to search for his questions, and to try to understand his story. I picked up some Cantonese—"jo san" was our morning greeting. I became associated with Mr. L. in the minds of the staff; I had them page me when he had the occasional visitor. I would hurry to his room, hoping in vain that this person could explain things to him more clearly or give me some special insight. I brought up Mr. L. during our inevitably speedy rounds, just to keep him from being summarized by the single word—"placement."

When I completed my medicine clerkship, Mr. L. had been in the hospital for over 8 weeks and continued to await placement. I said goodbye and told him I would no longer be taking care of him. He thanked me, and I believe he looked confused.

I don't know where Mr. L. is now, or how he is doing. I still think of him and wonder if we did right by him. I wonder if I did enough. I hope he has many visitors, and that he is greeted with "jo san" in the morning.

A Foreign Concept

RANJANA SRIVASTAVA, MBBS

The soft purr of the bedside telephone changes its cadence precipitously, and the shrill noise throws me out of my dream. Shaken out of a deep and tired sleep, I leap for the receiver.

"I am sorry, but there is an asthmatic girl who looks as if she will arrest. I have tried ..."

I slam the phone down; the other hand hastily scoops up my stethoscope, identification, and pen; I sprint to the emergency department, racing to beat the dire tones of the code siren that will resonate through the building at any moment.

I almost fall inside a cubicle, which holds an 18-year-old girl, heavily tattooed and excessively made up. She was out smoking marijuana when she felt the onset of an asthma attack. So she got one of her friends, an unlicensed driver, to rush her to the hospital. She is surrounded by a coterie of giggling teenagers, all looking remarkably fresh for the time of the night. It takes me a few moments to assess the situation.

"Stop hyperventilating," I say tersely to the patient. I turn to the others: "And all of you, get out now."

In silence, I finish my examination of the now subdued girl whose purported respiratory distress has dissipated to a mild wheeze. I stalk out of the cubicle, snatch a sheet of paper, and proceed to write emphatically in large script, double-spacing to stress my annoyance at this unceremonious awakening. The resident who called me stands penitently behind me.

"I am really sorry ..." he starts.

A chance glance at the clock, recollections of previous unnecessary calls, the thought of another long day ahead, and the sound of teenage mirth floating through the corridor provoke a surge of venom within me. Before I snap, I storm upstairs to my cold bed. The next morning, I receive a call from the same physician. The words tumble out before I have a chance to speak.

"The patient said she didn't want to see a doctor with an accent and then started acting very sick. I was afraid." Embarrassed and mollified by the explanation, I tell him to put the matter behind him.

A few weeks later, he timidly approaches me to help him practice for upcoming examinations to gain registration with the Australian Medical Council. Eager to restore amity, I readily agree. We start with common scenarios that candidates are examined on. I pretend to be an elderly diabetic whom he must counsel as my general practitioner. He makes a positive start, telling me what having the condition entails. He discusses optimal blood glucose levels and a healthy diet. He relaxes a little and hazards the advice that diabetes is not such a dangerous thing to have after all, then, ignoring the emerging doubt on my face, proceeds to tell me all about foot care.

"Your feet will become dead if you don't care."

"That sounds dangerous, Doctor," I hint.

"And you can get bad infections."

"Oh no!" I voice, in mock horror.

"And for that, you must prevent the crackles in your toys."

"*What?*"

"Ah, I will make you a picture." With a few deft strokes, he draws a shapely foot with a skin break between two toes. As he points proudly to his sketch, my pursed lips burst open with laughter.

"Crackles in the toys," he repeats, waving the paper into the air, puzzled by my response.

"Oh, oh, cracks in the *toes*, I mean," he corrects himself sheepishly.

"Let's start again," I say, grinning.

Weeks go by, and we continue to work on dozens of case studies. Sometimes I am the hypertensive, neurotic businessman; other times, a young woman with reflux. Sometimes I am the grateful and adherent patient; other times, the aggressive nightmare. Many of these sessions are dominated by criticism.

Mindful of the demands of my beeper, I can spend only short times tutoring, and I want to teach him much in the snatches of free time we have. So I press him to think about what the examiner wants, to prioritize information, show empathy, make eye contact, and say and do all the things that I determine he must bring naturally to these encounters if he is to pass.

Some days he is receptive; other days he cannot contain his woebegone expression. He wistfully mentions the great divide between my medical training and his own, but my beeper usually precludes elaboration. One day, he accompanies me to see a patient who has had a stroke. After assiduously examining the woman, I come unstuck at the constellation of neurologic signs that await a concise interpretation. While I gaze at the computed tomography scan of her brain, I suck on the end of my pen for inspiration.

A respectful voice appears at my side, "It is in the left cerebello-pontine junction."

I turn around, surprised.

"I used to be a neurosurgeon," he adds, almost apologetically.

At our next meeting, I put aside the demanding practice session in favor of finding out about the physician I teach but the person I barely know. A remarkable story unfurls before me.

The morning after a grueling night operating on a young girl injured in a terrorist attack, he woke up knowing he had to leave his homeland. Three months of unpaid salary aside, the guileless expression of his 5-year-old son sealed his conviction. He fled alone the next week, promising to find his wife and son a better life, secure from the drudgery of war.

Five years later, although he has discovered such a place, it has not proved easy for his family to immigrate. So he lives alone in the hospital quarters; the tenuous phone lines are his only link to the people left behind. His eyes shine as he speaks of his hopes for his son. Then I catch a glint behind his glasses, "I cannot forgive myself for not being there for my sister. She died during childbirth—I just wish I could have held her hand."

He could not return for her funeral for fear of being arrested. An unheralded image of my own family spread across continents crosses my mind, and I feel my throat constrict. Across the table, I sit still, entranced as the details of his existence emerge, like unshed rain, finally relenting. Suddenly, he makes a rising motion.

"I should let you go back to work."

I sense the aching urgency of unfinished business.

"Stay," I plead.

His father remains stoic about his son's move, but his ill mother's words of support are left stranded on her trembling lips when they speak. His wife frets, and the growing vagueness of his 10-year-old son over the phone hovers agonizingly over his days.

"It is as if he doesn't know his own father anymore."

A real fear of persecution, extending to his family, prevents him from returning home. So he holds on, with frail reserve, hoping for a better tomorrow. Neurosurgery seems a mere indulgence, once relished but now beyond the grip of circumstance. He is realistic about his options in a country that practices a different style of medicine.

He stares directly ahead for a few seconds as if summoning courage.

"You see, sometimes at work, I cannot forget about all these things, and I make bad calls to people like you because I don't think."

I am speechless. I feel like an impetuous storm, raging at an order of Nature it scarcely understands. Five years out of medical school, amid the heady days of youth and with the luxury of being able to gaze straight ahead without any real distractions to divert my focus, I have been blind to the trials that lash someone 15 years older, displaced from country, profession, and family, and straining to find a hint of solace in each passing day.

The hissing sound of the general dissatisfaction shared over the performance of many so-called foreign doctors echoes sorrily in my ears. For so many of them, the initial sweetness of escape has been soured by the bleakness of starting anew.

I feel his curious glance on me, awaiting my response.

"I had no idea" strikes me as a pathetic rejoinder to his cheerless tale.

So I ask him what I really want to: "Is the struggle worth it in the end?"

Unblemished radiance lightens his pensive expression.

"If my son lives to become a man and these struggles are just stories to tell his children, then … yes."

The beeper trills, demanding acknowledgment for its impeccable conduct over the last two hours. I have never been more grateful to hear its sound.

Postscript. Three months later, I received an exuberant call. He had passed the examinations with distinction.

A Little Confidence

ALAIN LE, BS

It was the second day of medical school and already we were headed up to the wards to confront our first real patients. With a shaking hand and a similar shake in my voice, I introduced myself as a first-year student. Sitting down in the chair beside my patient, I asked, "So, what brings you to the hospital today?" My inquisition steadily grew as more questions came pouring forth.

"How long has this been bothering you?

"Is there anything you do that makes the pain better?

"How has this illness affected your quality of life?"

Five minutes flew by in no time at all. Getting a patient history was a piece of cake, I thought. No sweat! Closing up the interview, I decided to ask my patient a simple question:

"Is there anything else I can do to help you with your stay?"

She replied, "Why, yes."

Wait! This was not going according to plan! In my role-playing activity just ten minutes earlier, my classmate had responded "No" to this same question. Already I could feel little beads of sweat starting to form on my forehead. What would she ask me? What kind of procedure could I possibly perform? What in the world could a student on his second day of medical school know that could possibly help any patient out? This was not fair; I was not yet trained to handle anything! I was 3 months away from studying the coagulation cascade, 12 months from learning the causes of hypoxemia, 25 months from understanding the management of gastrointestinal bleeding. In fact, I did not know medicine at all. Having graduating from college as a business major, I was a clean slate, devoid of medical knowledge.

Not knowing enough in medical school is something that frightens me every time I turn another page in the thousands that make up Cecil's *Textbook of Medicine*. I find myself repeating the phrases "I do not know" and "I did not know that" countless times each day. There is so much to learn, and I have been told that there will always be someone older and wiser telling me, "You still don't know anything yet." Indeed, it is hard to imagine that one can dedicate his or her entire life to medicine and still not know all there is to know. This is a humbling reality that I am going to have to get used to in this profession.

So there I was, sitting next to my patient bracing for her inevitable question. I realized the only thing that I could do at this point was to reach for something previously untested. Searching deep, I took hold of a little confidence. I was new, but eager, and there would be plenty of time to learn in the years to come. If I did not know the answer to her question, I would hold my head high and tell her that I could look it up or find someone who did know. Being confident in unexpected situations is something I would have to master if I wanted to become a good physician. Thus, I braced myself for this very first question that would test the limits of my medical knowledge. And so the patient asked me,

"Sir, could you turn the television back on when you leave?"

Harry James

LESLIE G. COHEN, MD

He was a lanky, crew-cut kid of 13, with a late-afternoon appointment to get refills for his asthma and acne medications. I had known him for a few years, so it was easy to pick up where we had left off 3 months before. After asking how he'd been since his last appointment, I briefly examined him, and wrote the prescriptions. Noticing his leather case on the floor, I asked, "Jesse, how long have you been playing the trumpet?"

"Two years now," he said, looking up. "The asthma doesn't bother me much."

"Do you take lessons?" I was interested.

"Yeah. It's tough finding time for everything, though. Next year I really want to learn how to play jazz." His eyes brightened.

"Do you play in the high school band?"

"Yep, the marching band. I wasn't good enough for the concert orchestra. Maybe next year," he smiled, his braces shining.

"You know, I used to play trumpet when I was your age. Pretty good, but not great," I said. "Have you ever listened to old recordings of Harry James?"

He shook his head, picked up the case, and walked to the door. With his hand on the doorknob, he turned, glanced at my diploma on the wall, then asked, "Tell me, how long does it take to be a doctor?"

I paused, then counted off the years for him, watching his face. He looked crestfallen. "Do you have good grades?" I asked hopefully.

"Yeah, real good, Doctor Cohen. School's not that hard."

"What do your parents think of your wanting to be a doctor?"

"They're not too happy with the idea. Too hard, they say."

"Never mind that, for now," I said. "I'm sure they'll come around in time. A high school teacher once told us to always follow our dreams. Listen, Jesse, my dad was a doctor and tried his damnedest to discourage me. I guess it made me try even harder. Keep up your good work. It is a very long road, but worth the trip. I hope you make it. See you in three months."

I sat at my desk for a few moments and closed my eyes, remembering a Sunday night over 40 years ago.

I had auditioned and qualified for a TV *Amateur Hour* sponsored by a local jewelry store. "E-Z Credit, E-Z Credit, Wilkens is the place where you can get it." Its jingle was fixed in my brain. My parents had stayed home to watch on our new DuMont.

I arrived at the television station just as the spotlights came on, and the six-piece band started playing the familiar theme music. The first contestant was an 8-year-old girl from Pittsburgh, who played "Blue Moon" very, very slowly on the saxophone. A few claps, probably her family. I felt sorry for the kid. Next, a pencil-thin schoolteacher from McKeesport faintly warbled "You'll Never Walk Alone." Inspirational—definitely a loser. Then it was my turn. "E-Z" Al Noble, the emcee with slick blonde hair and an on-camera smile, introduced me, and asked the usual questions. "Age?"

"13," I replied.

"School?"

"Taylor Allderdice Junior High School."

"Selection?"

" 'Body and Soul.' "

"What do you want to be when you grow up?"

"A doctor," I quickly replied, flashing a nervous smile.

The klieg lights made me sweat and blink. I shut my eyes and tried to stand tall. Pausing a second, I imagined the great Harry James, then smoothly played his jazzed-up version better than I'd ever practiced it. Loud applause from the studio audience startled me. I opened my eyes, amazed. Grinning and nodding, I took a seat off-stage.

I can't recall much about the rest of the show, except that a few weeks later I received a thank-you card in the mail stating that a polka band had the most mail-in votes. But what I vividly remember is my parents' welcome when I returned home. The door hadn't even closed when the inquisition began.

"You never told us you wanted to be a doctor," my mother snapped.

"I was afraid you'd think it was a silly idea, and be angry with me," I replied warily.

"With your big mouth you should be a lawyer," she replied. I just wanted to escape.

My father, the stern general practitioner, a man of few words—most of them sharp and critical—looked up from his newspaper. "Huh! You a doctor! You're too much of a lazy bum to be a doctor!" He solemnly turned back to the newspaper. Bitterly stung, I slowly walked up the stairs to my room.

The office buzzer sounded. I opened my eyes, teeth gritted, re-membering that grim time at home, and the difficult years that fol-lowed. Knowing Jesse's family, I felt sure they would support him in any path he chose. As I walked to the waiting room for my next pa-tient, I smiled, realizing I was whistling "Body and Soul."

Fake

JORDAN D. GRUMET, MD

With all the smugness of a physician
He stares at me
This fake

With glasses and clean-shaven face
Long white coat
Expensive tie
Pressed pants
Stethoscope wrapped around neck
And large name tag with small name next to big M and D

He searches me
With great confidence
For signs of
Weakness and frailty
Anxiety and insecurity
Disease and infirmity

But I see right through this fake
His quivering voice while answering superiors

His insecurity in the face of peers
His questioning of decisions about patients' well-being

And only I
Watch him belittle himself
Every morning
In front of my mirror
Before building enough courage
To leave his bedroom
And go to work

On Being a Patient

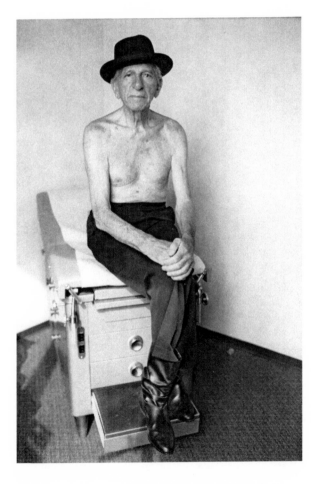

Scream

ELIZABETH BRODERICK, MD

"But you're a doctor." They don't say it, but it's in their eyes when I tell them that my husband was arrested for domestic assault and battery. My office manager tells me she doesn't understand it. She's told her husband that if he ever hits her he'd better make it a good one, because she's coming up off that floor and killing him. I tell her they don't start the relationship by hitting you.

At first, they are kind and loving and only trying to help you improve yourself. My husband would ask me medical questions: "I'm curious. How does this work?" I would explain, and he would start picking apart my answer. Eventually, he would ask me something I didn't know, and I would tell him I would have to look it up. Then he would say, "No, you don't need to do that," and I would feel stupid.

My patients certainly knew I had children. My pager would beep when I was on call, and I would get my messages and phone patients while simultaneously holding a child and fending off a screaming toddler grabbing my legs. My husband would read the paper in the family room. "I thought they would make even more noise if I took them away from you so I left them alone." I felt I wasn't doing a good job anywhere, as a mother, as a wife, as a physician. If I stayed late at work, he would call my cell phone.

"When are you coming home?"

"I have to finish my calls."

"Do them from here."

"I can't bring the charts home."

"The kids want you." The pressure never ended.

That night, I was screaming, "Leave me alone, leave me alone, leave me alone." He tried to slap me and I blocked him. He stepped forward, put one leg between mine, spun me in midair, and slammed me to the floor. I put my hands up over my head to show submission and curled sobbing into the fetal position. My right shin had slammed into a chair and was swollen and painful.

Then there was the shame of going to a local emergency room where they knew me. I had to tell them how my leg got hurt. I didn't know that the police would be called. I phoned my husband:

"The good news is, my leg isn't broken. The bad news is, you're going to be arrested."

After the police car slowly drove away, I walked through the house and looked at my sleeping children. I went into our room. I got into bed.

Don't scream.

Good girls don't scream.

A Road Less Traveled

HELEN W.

I kept buttoning and unbuttoning my black leather coat, responding to the alternating waves of heat and chill typical of narcotic withdrawal. It was a familiar sensation, but instead of being at home with the make-believe flu, I was sitting in a circle of fellow substance abusers sharing the misery and confusion of early sobriety.

We were a mixed bag of personalities, ages, ethnicities, income levels, and drugs of choice. There was a housewife who smoked pot daily, a young Filipino with a new baby and a methamphetamine habit, a 25-year-old blonde facing prison for her fifth DUI, an alcoholic ex-policeman showing signs of irreversible brain damage. And me: a middle-aged internist, mother, and narcotic addict.

I was the only doctor in that group, but I knew I wasn't unique. Nor was I treated with any particular deference. When my profession was discovered, a heroin user and recent prostitute sneered, "That's disgusting. You're supposed to help people. Anyway, you should know better."

I thought she was probably right.

There is never a simple explanation why someone becomes an addict. Spiritual deficits, character defects, low self-esteem, grandiosity, depression, bipolar disorder, obsessive-compulsive disorder, poor impulse control, genetic predisposition, childhood neglect or abuse: All have been implicated. But none of these causes addiction, though they may be contributing factors. For some people, a drink or a drug appears to be the answer to psychic discomfort. And it works, but only short term. There was a sense of revelation after my first dose of Percocet, which was prescribed after a dental extraction. I felt like Dorothy arriving in Oz. The world was suddenly a wonderful place. The usual anxieties and insecurities of a third-year medical student just starting clinical rotations were gone. I was a better, more confident me.

But I used narcotics intermittently, relying on legal, socially acceptable alcohol for taking the edge off after a hard day. Just about every night I was smoothed to the point of incoherence. I initially enjoyed my drinking, though usually I remembered little of it. Sometimes I'd have to piece it together with very few clues because I found people avoiding me after a festive evening. I believe I tended to offer my opinions loudly and repeatedly. Eventually I stopped drinking in public since once I got started, anything might happen. Besides, it was easier to sleep it off if I was already home, and I didn't have to struggle for the right to drive my own damn car.

But I could always work, through blinding hangovers, nausea, and fatigue, only to do it all again whenever I could. Valium with my morning coffee helped get me through the shaky morning after. I lived for my own private happy hour at the end of the day: several drinks before, during, and after a hasty dinner, then passing out in bed, sometimes still fully clothed. Most addicts and alcoholics become fairly adept at covering up the signs and symptoms of their disease. I would sneak bottles in and out of the house in my purse, rotate my purchases at various neighborhood stores, and dump the empty bottles in public trashcans. Vodka, of course, chased by a beer or two. Only after the birth of my children (I did quit drinking during pregnancy) did I switch to narcotics, as alcohol-induced blackouts made me an unfit mother. I was diagnosed with postpartum depression after my husband found me home alone with the children and barely responsive. "Socially," I lied, when the psychiatrist asked about my alcohol consumption. "Antisocially" would have been accurate. I hid my drinking so well that even my husband didn't realize the true nature of my affliction.

When I started to use narcotics, it seemed like the answer to my alcohol problems. It was portable and odorless. No confusing blackouts or loss of emotional control. I didn't stagger, and I could drive with no need to close one eye. I could even drink "normally" while using narcotics, although I never understood why anyone would want to. At work, the pills helped me stay calm and focused amidst the chaos, and if my drug abuse was suspected, I was never confronted with it. For awhile it seemed I had it all under control, until one day I realized that I was not "in control" at all. I thought the drugs were helping me live my life, but, like a voracious parasite, they had taken over my life. I lived to obtain and use narcotics.

Go to a few AA meetings and, if you're like me, you'll hear your own story over and over again. The illusion, the crash, the "incomprehensible demoralization." You'll find that all of your "clever" ruses to obtain your drug of choice were fairly mundane and that others were much more creative. Like the woman who rifled medicine cabinets at open houses. The actors who feign migraines, toothache, or back pain: the bane of every emergency department. Addiction-prone doctors have such easy access to narcotics that cleverness and acting skills aren't necessary. After awhile, ethics and morality and legal sanctions seem meaningless compared with our compelling need. Toward the end of my drug use, my life revolved around getting more.

Stopping the escalating cycle of addiction first required a moment of clarity. One day I understood that there was no end in sight and that to continue would require too much. Too much risk, too much time and energy, too much of my life. There was no euphoria anymore, merely the staving off of withdrawal. I was at the end of the road, but I couldn't stop on my own. So I picked up the phone, called the "physician well-being committee," and found myself in that diverse circle, sharing personal issues with people I'd never met before. There I realized that I was no better and no worse than any of them. By sharing our humanity we could start to become human again.

That's when I started on that long and winding road back to Kansas. There are no ruby slippers involved, just lots of meetings, bad coffee, stale pastry, and friends made and lost. Three members of that initial recovery group have died of their addictions. We survivors mourned them but also tried to understand why. Perhaps then we could save ourselves.

There's no magic formula for recovery. I'm part of the physician's diversion program, so I get random urine tests and monitoring at weekly peer-support meetings. When recovery had not yet consolidated into a way of life, random testing and daily naltrexone use were effective relapse deterrents. Twelve-step groups help many people, although some balk at their religious overtones and "higher power" concept. Therapy, with or without medication, can help. Some of us need to "change everything"; others need minor adjustments.

The only universal truth is, we can't drink or use drugs ever again.

I had used alcohol and drugs in response to almost any situation: to change a bad mood, enhance a good one, alleviate tedium, or no reason at all. Unlike many others in recovery, I have no major psychiatric disorder, childhood trauma, or other deep psychological wounds to recover from as well. But long-term use of mind-altering substances tends to stunt emotional growth.

In sobriety I need to develop healthy coping strategies and learn to cultivate serenity. I now realize I can deal with any situation more effectively and more creatively when sober, but change is slow. At work I take "one patient at a time," try to stay centered, and have a phone list of supporters to provide perspective if I'm losing mine. Sometimes when I feel stressed or depressed or angry, I still want that artificial escape. But in recovery, feelings have lost their power. I don't deny them, but neither do I feel the need to react to them. And they pass.

The main reason I stay sober is that the alternative is simply not worth it. I accept that I'm not capable of "normal" drinking and if I relapsed, I could lose my job, my license, my self-esteem, my family, and even my life. Obviously (from a sober vantage point) nothing is worth that risk.

Every day I realize how many wonderful experiences are available without need of chemical enhancement: playing with my children, talking to patients, chatting with colleagues, going to the gym, strong coffee, good books, music, a sound night's sleep. It's an endless list of pleasures, whereas previously I had only one.

I have increased awareness of addiction and alcohol problems in my practice, although they are difficult to diagnose through layers of isolation, fear, shame, and denial. Sharing personal stories is a large part of how AA works; newcomers recognize that they are not alone, that their worst behavior is not unique, and that recovery is possible. Although I feel an affinity for those who struggle, I rarely reveal my history to patients. Instead I reach out to "the alcoholic who still suffers" with empathy and understanding.

Maybe that's the reason I traveled that road myself.

Editor's Note: Helen W. is a pseudonym.

Stuck

CHRISTINE SEIBERT, MD

I felt a brief prick on the pad of my right third finger. I did not say or do anything to alert the resident with whom I was working, but instead continued until the lumbar puncture on our patient with end-stage AIDS was finished. Then I stared at my glove before taking it off, putting it in a bag and then in my pocket so I could scrutinize it later, without arousing suspicion. I examined my finger and there was no puncture, no gash, and no blood. While I meticulously scrubbed my hands, I debated whether or not to call Employee Health. It was 11:45 P.M. and I was tired. I had a desperate urge to go home, kiss my kids, long asleep, and climb into bed with my husband. I did not want to make a big deal out of this in the middle of the night.

After my drive home, I walked in the house and scrubbed my hands again. Then I doused them with bleach for good measure, not remembering whether or not this was helpful. I crept into my daughters' rooms to complete our nightly parental ritual of checking on each of them before going to bed. I do not know how long I stood and stared at them, wondering whether our lives would ever be the same again.

I awoke the next morning with a deep dread. From home, I called a friend who is an infectious disease consultant, luckily on service that month. I related my story to him, and he sprang into action, swiftly arranging for me to be seen first thing that morning in Employee Health to get a dose of zidovudine and lamivudine. He first admonished me for not calling him sooner. But he must have sensed the mounting panic in my voice and kindly reassured me that I did not do irrevocable harm with my delay. Later he met me for lunch, armed with what seemed like the world's literature on needlestick injuries in health care workers. Gently, he recited the statistics and reported that my risk for seroconversion was 3 in 1000. He was encouraged. I had been hoping for one in a million.

After recounting the details of my exposure again, he recommended 30 days of prophylactic drug therapy. Grateful for any ammunition to ward off HIV, I agreed that I could take any concoction for a month if it would stack the deck in my favor. Before deciding which drugs to take, my friend suggested that I meet with another expert in this area. Though I was leery of telling anyone else, I allowed my friend to make the arrangements.

The expert paged me that evening. I met him at his HIV clinic, feeling self-conscious immediately upon walking through the door. In one of the exam rooms, I told my story again. Though his work in the hospital was not done and it was already 6 P.M., the expert was patient, thorough, and sympathetic. I will always be grateful that I shared my secret with him. He decided on a three-drug combination of zidovudine, lamivudine, and nelfinavir, one of the newer protease inhibitors. I would feel like I had the flu and would have a significant chance of diarrhea. He gave me pointers on how to prevent the diarrhea by eating Metamucil bars along with twice-daily calcium. He tactfully reviewed how to protect my husband and family. I added condoms to my mental grocery list.

I left the clinic with my prescriptions and strategized how and where I would fill them with the least wagging of tongues. The pharmacy where my husband works was out, as was my neighborhood pharmacy. I decided on the seemingly anonymous hospital pharmacy. When I brought my prescriptions to the window, the pharmacist looked at my white coat, then at the prescriptions again and asked,

"Are these for you?" I replied affirmatively, causing her to quickly avert eye contact and awkwardly busy herself. After the prescriptions were filled, I was nervous when I saw a familiar face at the pick-up window. The pharmacist and I exchanged pleasantries, and he admirably hid most of his surprise at the drugs I was getting. I felt compelled to explain my story to him so he would not judge me as I felt the other pharmacist had done. He wished me luck in a pitying sort of way. I nearly ran back to my office.

There was still one more task before heading home. I had to have baseline labs drawn. Knowing how vulnerable a computerized record can be, I asked the Employee Health nurse to allow me to have my labs drawn under an alias. I shed my not-so-anonymous white coat in my office and reluctantly walked toward the lab with my requisition. I got questioning looks from the check-in person, as well as from my tactless phlebotomist, who asked me why I was getting my blood drawn with an alias. I explained that I was an employee and I wanted to keep my medical care private. That produced the same aversion of gaze I experienced earlier at the pharmacy counter.

Finally at home, my girls gave me their customary welcome mauling and then ran into the backyard to finish some sandbox creations. As soon as I made eye contact with my husband, I burst into tears. He tried to comfort me, but I would have none of it. The events of the day and my own imaginings of the worst possible conclusions to this incident squashed my usual optimism.

That night, when putting my daughters to bed, I hugged them tighter and longer than usual, crying silently as I lay down with each of them that evening. I imagined how HIV would affect my family. I calculated how old they would be when I would begin to suffer the ravages of the disease. Would I embarrass them? Would I be a burden? Would they forget how vital and energetic I used to be? As tears streamed down my face in the darkness while I hugged my youngest, I was immediately taken aback. What was the concentration of HIV in human tears? I quickly let her go, jumped out of bed, and ran out of the room to wash my hands and face.

The first week after my needlestick was the hardest. Already worn out from nearly a month of being the ward attending, I began to feel increasingly achy and sluggish. My eyelids seemed to gain 20 pounds as I uncharacteristically fought to keep them open at every conference or meeting. I became hypervigilant about touching my family. One evening after I absentmindedly licked my fingers before rubbing some debris off of my daughter's cheek, I became nauseated with dread after realizing my mistake. This new obsessive antiseptic approach was going to be hard on our family of lackadaisical hand washers, who seemed to share a lot of body fluid, not to mention the occasional toothbrush.

Over the next few weeks, I played more and worked less, coming home much earlier than usual. I noticed the blooming zinnias in my backyard and started cutting them for arrangements. My husband and I began taking long walks after dinner. I joined my daughters' tea parties and swung with them on their swing set. I read few, if any journals, instead focusing my efforts on novels I always wanted to read. I did not exercise as much, partly from exhaustion and partly because it did not seem to matter. I became impatient with patients who came in with "trivial" concerns. Time was wasting, after all.

The next milestone was my first follow-up HIV test. I was not bothered as much about the inquisitive looks at the lab this time. After a month of the three-drug regimen, I was spent. How did people take those toxins month after month? I hoped I was not going to find out. For several days after my test, I got a sick feeling in my chest every time I was paged to a number I did not immediately recognize, sure I was going to get bad news. About a week later, a letter from the hospital came for me at home. Though I was fairly sure that positive results would not be sent in the mail, I made my husband open the envelope. I finally exhaled after finding out I had dodged the bullet that time.

During the next few months, I searched my soul and reprioritized my life. I became a better mom and wife, a more empathetic doctor, and a more caring friend. Like Sleeping Beauty, my life changed with the prick of a finger. I was now holding out for the fairy tale ending.

One in Three

DAVID MALEBRANCHE, MD, MPH

A few years ago, the Centers for Disease Control and Prevention reported that one out of every three black men who have sex with men are HIV positive. Since I am a physician who happens to be both black and homosexual, I belong to this risk group. For me, getting an HIV test is a yearly ritual—it's something many black men who have sex with men do because of the fear embedded in our psyches for simply being who we are.

During my latest doctor's visit, a nurse drew my blood and told me to return for my test results in a week. I left with the usual amount of anxiety that accompanies an HIV test, keenly aware of my "risk group" status. One week later, I returned to the clinic, and after I waited for what seemed to be two hours (although in reality it was only thirty minutes), a nurse informed me that my test results had not yet returned.

Physicians make horrible patients. We dismiss physical symptoms altogether, or we give ourselves the most serious diagnosis possible. If we urinate frequently, it's diabetes. A mole is melanoma; a persistent cough, tuberculosis. I work at an HIV clinic, so I know that HIV serum antibody tests are actually a series of three tests (two enzyme-linked immunosorbent assays [ELISAs] and one Western blot test). If the first ELISA is negative, the result will be in the computer within two days. After a week, if the test results are not in, it's likely that the first ELISA result is positive and the lab is confirming the diagnosis with the second ELISA and the Western blot. Knowing this and being told my HIV test was pending after a week was not a good thing. But the nurse shrugged her shoulders and just smiled at me.

"Why don't you come back in a couple days? It should be ready by then," she said.

"Well, it's been a week, and it shouldn't be longer unless something's wrong, right?" I said.

"Unfortunately we don't have the results yet. I'm sorry."

I left with a polite "thank you."

At home, I revisited my sexual experiences from the past year, including my inconsistent condom use. I looked for rashes and lymph nodes and examined every crevice of my body for anything suggesting HIV infection. I found nothing, but the Centers for Disease Control and Prevention says I'm at risk because of who I am, and in my heart I knew I was at risk for what I had done. I thought, "*Could I become the next one-in-three statistic on the pages of medical journals and in media headlines? I can see it now—the HIV doctor who couldn't practice what he preached.*"

Two days passed, and I returned to the doctor's office for my test results. In the waiting room, I hoped to have the nurse I had spoken to before. She had a benevolent demeanor that puts you at ease like you're home with your mama.

"Mr. Malebranche," a loud voice called. Another nurse, heavier in weight and attitude, led me into a cold examining room and left. It was 10:00 A.M.

Five minutes later, the nurse returned and handed me a paper.

"You're negative. Everything looks good," she said.

I saw the syphilis test result. "Nonreactive," it read. Good. Further down, I saw the HIV antibody test result. "In laboratory," it read. I choked on my own breath.

"What about the HIV test?" I asked.

"It's negative," she said flatly.

"No it's not. It's still in the laboratory. Why isn't it back yet?" I asked.

She took the paper from me and looked at it.

"You're right. Why don't you come back in a couple of days? It should be back then," she said.

A couple of days? Again? My blood boiled as I tried to remain calm despite the nonchalant style in which she was providing me with HIV-test counseling. *"I can't be the stereotypical angry black man—not now,"* I thought.

"Ma'am, I'm a physician. I do work with HIV. I know what it means when an HIV test takes a long time to come back. Could you call the lab to find out, please?"

Half recognizing my fear and half annoyed by my insistence, she reluctantly exited. My mind remained on one horrific thought: *"This is it. I'm HIV positive."*

Although I know HIV is not a death sentence, that cliché was more difficult to swallow when I thought about my own HIV status. I looked at the clock—10:10 A.M. I thought about my HIV-positive friends whom I would call first for support. 10:20 A.M. How would I tell my family? Parents aren't supposed to bury their children. 10:30 a.m. *"I need to tell my recent sexual partners so they can get tested as well,"* I thought. 10:40 A.M. Beads of sweat trickled down my forehead as my heart beat out of my chest. *So this is what a panic attack feels like.*

10:55 A.M. The nurse with the benevolent demeanor entered, and I couldn't remember ever being so happy to see a familiar face in my entire life. She smiled at me.

"Hey, you were here the other day for your test results. You get them yet?" she asked.

"No, but one of the other nurses left me here at ten o'clock to check on my HIV test—it's still listed as 'In laboratory.'"

"Do you remember the nurse's name?"

"No, but she's heavyset."

She looked at me curiously. Something was wrong.

"What is it?"

"Well, we only have one heavyset nurse here, and she just went on her lunch break."

"She went on lunch break?!"

"Yeah. Listen, baby, I'll go check on those results for you myself. I'll be right back."

I was furious. How could a medical professional take a lunch break and leave a patient waiting for HIV test results, especially when the patient is a physician who has explained his anxiety to her? Maybe she didn't know that I belong to a "risk group" or inconsistently used condoms, and thus didn't prioritize my test results over her eating. *"If she treats fellow medical personnel like this, how does she treat other patients?,"* I thought. My body was numb. *"This is it—I'm HIV positive."*

11:00 A.M. After I'd spent a full hour in that sterile examining room, the benevolent nurse returned.

"The lab faxed the results. I just have to get one of the doctors to sign off on it, and you can go home," she said.

As thankful as I was, the benevolent nurse was still missing the most important part of this whole interaction.

"The results?!" I said impatiently.

"Oh, it's negative."

She handed me a paper, which shook in my trembling hand. Below my name, next to "HIV antibody test," it said "Negative." I started to cry.

"Why was it still listed as 'In laboratory' if it was negative?" I asked.

"I don't know, honey, these things happen. I'm sorry you were put through this."

"That's OK." But I was lying to her. I wasn't OK. I handed the paper back to her, wiping the tears from my eyes.

"Could you please make a copy of this for me?" I needed written confirmation of the bullet I had just dodged.

"No problem."

As she left, I wanted to take my frustration out on the nurse who had deserted me, but that would have been displaced. She didn't put me at risk for HIV. I did.

Maybe being a black homosexual man isn't my real HIV risk group, but being a physician is. We often advise our patients to engage in healthy behavior, yet frequently we smoke tobacco and drink alcohol, have poor nutritional habits, and have unprotected sex as if we are immune to disease ourselves. A colleague of mine recently informally surveyed several medical professionals regarding HIV-test practices. She found that many have unprotected sex, but the only ones who were routinely tested were homosexual men and pregnant women. She asked me, "Does our status affect us knowing our status?"

Often, medical personnel don't follow proper HIV-testing and counseling practices. People sometimes avoid HIV tests because of past negative medical experiences and fear of the testing process. Now I see why. If we discourage people with our approach to HIV testing and counseling, individuals and communities will continue to go untested, those with HIV will not know their status, and the epidemic will continue.

The benevolent nurse returned with a copy of my test results. "I hope this doesn't prevent you from coming back here for your next test," she said.

But I knew that I would never go back to that office again.

I was too emotionally drained to wait for the "lunch-break nurse" to return and chastise her in person. A life awaited me where my status as a physician or a black homosexual man didn't influence my HIV-risk assessment, but rather encouraged me to engage in safer sex and get tested on the basis of my behavioral risk. I stepped outside to a glorious summer morning, no longer fooling myself about my risk for contracting a disease simply because of who I am.

One in three? Not if I have anything to say about it.

Inventory

RAE VARCOE, MA, MB, ChB

this is my bed
these are my sheets
here is my clock
on unsteady locker

my pillow fixes my scalp
restraining my
fears from flight
my thoughts turn in

in the locker are my books
my hands, too weak
to hold them now
hold instead, your hand

the morphine comes
between me and thought
between me and pain
between you and me

the nurses do not say
how long, or when
the god who might say why
has long since gone

this is my bed
this is my body
this is my life
these are my letters

Nightmare from the Sixties

PENELOPE J. TIPTON

Even after 30 years, it remains difficult for me to tell this story. And if doctors can learn from it, then I suppose the story is worth the telling.

I was at the time a college student in Boston. It was in those days of the sixties, those days of the Beatles and Vietnam, when protest was everywhere—and yet, incredibly, the Brahmins of Boston, together with the Catholic Church, still managed to legislate morality. Having myself been sheltered from life by family and Church, I found the freedom of the university setting exciting, and—I won't make excuses—I found the intimacies of sex too inviting to resist. In other words, I learned at that time in my life what is now for many teenagers common experience in high school.

Birth control was illegal in Massachusetts in those days. One purchased the Pill or condoms across the border or used "the rhythm method," as the Church fathers had instructed. As if passion can be planned.

I became pregnant.

These were the days, remember, when there were no clinics one might call upon anonymously—no Planned Parenthood, no understanding physicians readily at hand. Abortion was illegal and, where it was illegally practiced, a danger to one's life. "Don't go the coathanger route," was the piece of advice my sensitive roommate tossed to me on her way out the door one Saturday night. And from my chemistry laboratory partner came another: "Potassium permanganate, those purple crystals used in indicator solutions for qualitative analysis lab, can induce a spontaneous abortion." "It is," she had whispered, "an abortifacient."

I stole the jar of crystals from the chemistry lab and, in the privacy of my room, removed about a third of the contents, and then replaced the jar on the shelf in the lab before anyone could notice it missing. But how did one use the stuff? It came without instructions. Just the red label—"poisonous"—on the jar. Well, then, not by mouth, certainly. Douche with a solution of the crystals? No, probably not concentrated enough; and it would all simply drain out, sort of, before it could work. So, I supposed, just get enough of the crystals deep into the vagina. Using a cardboard tube from a tampon together with a make-shift funnel, I inserted the cylinder as deeply into my vagina as its length would allow, and then poured about a third of the bottle of crystals into the paper funnel. Down the tube they rattled. I could feel them settle deep inside. I felt all at once apprehensive, desperate, and cheap. Can you possibly know that feeling?

Potassium permanganate is an oxidizer. Read—*corrosive*; read—*pain*. Within 10 minutes, the pain had me doubled over. In 20, I was screaming for help out into the dorm corridor. In 45, I was in the emergency room. By then, I was physically ill with the pain, out of my head with my predicament—crying, sobbing, and screaming, uncontrollably, and all at once. There I was—National Merit Scholar, "all-American home-town kid," my parents' pride and joy, "Daddy's little girl"—lying on a stretcher in a hospital with my pregnant uterus and my self-inflicted vaginal burns.

The nurses were busy. They were, as I remember, concerned. One even seemed frightened. But mostly, they were busy. The first physician who came—I guessed he was an emergency room physician—never looked at me, never greeted me, never touched me. He looked somewhere at a spot on the wall and said,

"Vaginal bleeding? Call G-Y-N."

After an eternity, after an intravenous, after three blood pressures had been taken, and after five "it-won't-be-long"s, the gynecology resident finally came in.

"Get me some light," he said. "Let's get her legs up and spread 'em." Oh, the wonderful soul-connecting intimacy of the physician–patient relationship! But I didn't care. I wanted relief from the pain. I wanted a safe place to go to. I just wanted to be cared for.

"Think I'm stupid?" said the resident.

"I'm sorry?" I asked.

"You think I'd fall for this? Christ, what a sorry broad!" he said to no one in particular, and left. I had been there on the stretcher in the ER now for over an hour, still no relief from the pain. I was later to learn that the corrosive crystals had perforated my vagina. He left me, this doctor, with my feet in stirrups, my knees spread, the curtain to the room open, and my pudenda exposed to the world passing by. Soon he returned with another young man. I was too sick with the pain to look at either of them, to study and learn their faces, but I will never forget their voices.

"Stick your fingers in there, stud," said the resident, "and learn what a gravid uterus feels like."

"No," said the medical student.

"No? Whaddya mean 'no'? You've gotta learn from this! This bitch thought that by inducing *vaginal* bleeding with a corrosive, she might trick me into thinking it was *cervical* bleeding. Then I'd perform a D and C and she'd have her abortion. Well, no deal. Stick your fingers in there and do a bi-manual."

"No, I can't do that," said the medical student. "I just can't do that."

"Listen, pal," said the resident, "You wanna scrub in? You want a decent call schedule? You want a good evaluation? You do what I tell you to do!"

"No, I'm sorry," said the student. He looked at me. Our eyes caught, and for the briefest of moments, my pain was secondary. He was not about to add to my humiliation. He had tears in his eyes. "I'm sorry," he said to me. Then he left.

In the process of the repair of the perforation and its aftermath, I had a spontaneous abortion. I will tell you now—30 years later—because I have a feeling you might wonder, that I have three daughters and that I have talked to them about this experience.

I'll give you no moral lecture about "choice" or "right to life," no invective against the Church and "the Laws of Men," who legislate a morality of their own liking. But I will tell you this. I hope that medical student became a physician, because it seems to me your profession needs people like that.

Palpation

NANCY FITZ-HUGH MENEELY

It's not my fingers haven't told me
truths about a summer honeydew,

the underside of leaves
and warmth retained in the evening's lake.

It's not they wouldn't understand
the need to move like whispering

beneath my daughter's hair,
around my husband's mouth.

But when I make them probe
the complex privacy of my breast

invade its unresisting slide
across the mooring of my bones

my fingers are clumsy and reckless,
carnival seers foretelling my chances

of grief, romance, longevity,
declaring tragedy from mere abundance

or hurrying past some grain of truth
too hard to understand.

I'd rather let them gather into comfort
underneath this density of flesh, hold me

in suspense and tell the simpler story
of my weight and heat, passivity.

Dr. Mommy Blues

GALE BURSTEIN, MD, MPH

One rather dreary morning during my fellowship, I walked into clinic to find the nurses hovered in a corner, intensely whispering. Always keen to uncover department scandal, I approached the group to get the news. Bubbling with the anticipation of a juicy piece of gossip, I asked, "Hey, ladies, what's the word today?" Instead of the rush of giggles that usually followed this question, sad stares from eyes welled with tears focused on me. "A second-year Ob-Gyn resident who had a 6-month-old jumped off the roof of the parking garage and killed herself this morning," flatly relayed one of the nurses.

How terrible, but why didn't this young woman ask someone for help? How could that happen? We are the vestige of a nationally recognized academic medical center. Our institution has a plethora of social workers, psychologists, and psychiatrists. She worked in a department where faculty should be wearing antennas programmed to find and destroy postpartum depression. How could they miss postpartum depression in their own resident? What magnitude of sadness and despair could drive a mother to leave her newborn baby? As a young girl, I frequently asked that question—"How could this happen?"—only to hear, "You will understand when you are older." Since

I was now a board-certified pediatrician and still did not understand, I assumed that I never would. Little did I know.

Seven years later I am a productive medical researcher at a large federal agency, wife of an assistant professor of medicine at an acclaimed medical academic center, and mother of two boys. Sounds great, right? Appearances can be deceptive.

My oldest son had several chronic medical and behavioral problems that gnawed away our resilience. Although my second son, 6 months old, was a healthy and beautiful baby, things were not going well. My milk supply was dwindling. I was not enjoying my children and was very anxious about the prospect of spending time alone with them. I had difficulty sleeping and loss of appetite.

Work was another world. I was very productive, publishing manuscripts and submitting book chapters. Colleagues praised me for successfully juggling a family and a career and marveled at my ability to lose all my postpartum weight so quickly. Work was the only place where I felt in control. But this world ended at 5:00 P.M. every day and did not exist on weekends.

I found myself asking questions like, "How can I keep doing this? Will this ever end?" Wishing away my sons' childhoods, desperate to run away from my failed attempts at motherhood, I searched for an answer. I remembered that obstetrics–gynecology resident who had jumped off the roof of a six-story parking garage. I now understood her desperation. But I also understood that I had kids who needed me. Although I was not anticipating a nomination for Mother of the Year, I still truly believed that nobody could love or care for my sons like I could. No question. I had to be there for them, which meant I had to get help.

I made numerous phone calls, but I could not maneuver my way through my health care system to obtain authorization for mental health services. Horrified at the prospect of calling another stranger to explain that I was crazy and needed psychiatric care, I resorted to calling the human resources management office at work. I spoke to an angel who gave me the phone number that saved me. Although I could not get an appointment with a psychiatrist for several days, just knowing that I would soon get care allowed me to go through the motions of getting out of bed in the morning, going to work, talking to my family at dinner, and going to sleep.

My psychiatrist appointment was scheduled for 4:30 on the afternoon of September 11, 2001. Nothing could make me miss that appointment.

In the psychiatrist's office, I manically lamented about my anhedonia. My psychiatrist listened with a blank stare. After a few minutes, he ordered me to stop speaking and proclaimed, "You are *wired*." He wrote a prescription for an antidepressant with an anxiolytic effect and advised me to return in two weeks for follow-up and medication adjustment. I made an *a priori* decision to be a compliant patient. The stakes were too high, my knowledge of psychopharmacology was too low, and I desperately wanted to experience happiness again.

Slowly I returned to life. After a few weeks of treatment and a higher medication dose, I was not afraid to spend time with my kids. After a few more weeks of treatment and another medication dose increase, I *enjoyed* being with my kids. Then, after several months, I *loved* hanging out with my kids again. I was finally able to thoroughly appreciate my family. I happily fed my youngest son formula instead of breast milk. My oldest son was making substantial improvements in his health and behavioral status. I even continued to be productive at work. Yes, life was good again. After 6 months of treatment, I proclaimed to my psychiatrist that I was ready to try life without medication. One month later, I was antidepressant-free and have not looked back ... until today.

Today is my one-year anniversary of my last dose of antidepressant. I feel so fortunate that I was able to get help and not suffer the fate of a peer from long ago. In my dreams, I reach out to her. If I had been in her shoes, a new mom, a resident consumed by call, sleep deprivation, long work days, little time off from work, and little income, would I have found my way to help?

Although our medical profession communicates to patients that mental health should not be stigmatized, we are guilty of that very stigmatization. From now on, in every application for employment, hospital privileges, and malpractice insurance, I will be expected to check the box that asks if I have ever received psychiatric care or counseling without being offered the opportunity to explain those circumstances or affirm that I am "cured."

Before my own experience with postpartum depression, I was guilty of assuming those same stereotypes. Knowing what I know today, I wonder why I had those beliefs. I wonder why more physicians are unable to be sympathetic to their colleagues' harsh realities of new motherhood, which add to their already high baseline stress level. I wonder why more physicians do not thoughtfully suggest to an unhappy new-mother colleague that she may benefit from mental health services. I wonder why I ponder the possibility of being denied a job, hospital privileges, or malpractice insurance if I check the box on the application that categorizes me as someone with a psychiatric history. I wonder why I have to think twice about signing my name to this essay. I wish I did not have to ask these questions. I hope other physicians wish the same.

Free Fall

GENA KAY McKINLEY, MD

"Mrs. M., the doctor is here to see you."

I looked up to see a nurse peering sympathetically at me.

"Huh?" I thought. "But *I'm* the doctor. Where am I?"

I looked around. I was on a single mattress on the floor in an other-wise empty green room. "A quiet room?!" I thought. I didn't feel quiet. Why couldn't I be still? What's wrong with my legs? I sat up on the mattress and kept shaking my feet. A doctor was crouched down on a stool with a nurse standing beside him.

"Umm, Mrs. M.," she said, making a "cross your heart" gesture of modesty for me to cover my breasts.

What the heck? I had a robe with nothing to tie it together? What's that about?

"Right, right." I closed my shirt but my feet wouldn't stay still.

"Mrs. M., do you know where you are?" the doctor asked.

"Uh-oh," I thought. It's a Mini-Mental Status! Where was I? I was in a hospital, yes, but not *my* hospital. This wasn't one of our doctors! Who were these people?

"Mrs. M.," the nurse said again, making the little motion for me to cover my breasts. I had already forgotten.

"Well, let me see," I said. I kept wriggling and looking around. "I'm not really sure where I am."

"What do you remember?" the doctor asked.

"I remember the nausea. I hate nausea." I started to cry.

"How long did you have nausea?"

"About a year," I said. To say it out loud made me feel foolish.

"What happened with the nausea that got you here?" he pushed further.

"My stomach had been bothering me a lot but I thought it was in my head. I've been under a lot of stress." A bad divorce, single parenting, a difficult practice—why wouldn't my stomach bother me? I knew that I was *Helicobacter pylori*–positive, so I asked a colleague to treat me for it. But the nausea was driving me crazy. I asked him for metoclopramide because the other anti-nausea medications made me too sleepy.

"I got the Reglan, and I took one dose and another dose the next morning. I remember feeling very restless by the time I saw my first patient. I thought it was the Reglan, but since you need to take it four times a day, I figured I wouldn't take any more and I'd be fine."

"Then what happened?"

"I remember telling a patient that I felt funny, and I kept dropping things. I didn't get better as the day wore on. My mind felt frozen. I made it through most of my day but cancelled my last appointment. I thought I'd go to bed early and that the next day whatever it was would be gone. I remember thinking, 'I'll go to sleep, I'll wake up, and it will be gone.' "

"Were you better when you woke up?"

"No. I wasn't better; I was worse. I was frightened, and I couldn't be still for two seconds. I had no idea what was wrong with me. I was no longer a doctor. I was just a patient who *needed* a doctor. I called my friend who had prescribed the Reglan. I told him that I couldn't be still, that my muscles hurt. I was scared. I thought I was going crazy. I begged him to help me."

"What did your colleague do?"

"He came over and said he didn't know what was wrong with me. I was frantic. The Reglan had me in a complete headlock. I called my psychiatrist and got voice mail. I left a message that she had to help me; something was badly wrong. I made my colleague drive me to see her. I writhed around in a total state of panic until she was free. I told her what I was taking, and she recognized my symptoms instantly as akathisia from the Reglan. Somewhere in my brain I had memories of inpatient treatment with IV Benadryl and people ministering to the agitation. I would be okay. I had to let go and trust that I would be taken care of."

"Were you admitted then?" The doctor pushed back his chair with his hiking boots.

"No, I wasn't. Instead of being sent to the hospital, I was given a prescription for Valium, which my colleague had filled for me. He drove me home and dropped me off. I don't remember much from the days that followed until I woke up in here. I don't know who took care of my son."

"That's quite a story. How do you feel now?"

"I feel like bugs are crawling under my skin and I want to tear it off," I said, to my own amazement.

"We'll try to keep you from doing that, and we'll give you some medicine to keep you calmed down. I'll check on you later." The doctor and his entourage left me. I was alone in my "quiet" room.

Eventually, things do wash out, even the haloperidol that was given to me before I was shipped to this hospital via Lear jet—the haloperidol that had worsened my akathisia and dystonia considerably. I now know from reviewing my records that this home remedy for akathisia didn't go too well. My records report that I was prescribed more diazepam, which I had to pick up at a pharmacy, wrecking my car in the process. I was given lorazepam and other medications that agitated me further. At some point I had been walked over to the house of the psychiatrist and had been given secobarbital. None of this was effective. I completely lost my faculties. Before my transfer I had started to break things, and the psychiatrist finally decided to admit me to the hospital. Now, though, my admission was involuntary because I had become psychotic from the cocktail of medications given to me over the past three or four days.

I learned that assault charges had been filed against me by the police who brought me to the hospital. My involuntary limb movements and impaired cognition had been perceived as attempts at assault. The charges made newspaper headlines. I was investigated by the state medical board. Can you imagine the personal cost?

Here is the belief that this nightmare has reinforced in me. We need to care for ourselves and for our fellow physicians in the same way that we take care of our patients. As hard as it is for us physicians to let go of complete control and to submit to being a *patient*, we need to trust that, when we do, our colleagues will be there: ready, willing, and able to take care of us with the same degree of skill, compassion, and dignity that we ourselves give to those we treat.

A Visit to the Doctor

DEBORAH YOUNG BRADSHAW, MD

The door opened without resistance, and I entered. The doctor's waiting room was decorated with the popular industrial plums, blues, and grays, but there was enough mahogany to impart a sense of reverence. The room was tasteful yet warm, and it reassured me. I was surprised to be greeted there by a patient of my own, a doctor himself. It was like looking into a mirror, with doctor doctoring doctor, doctoring doctor, receding into infinity. My patient was an elderly man, a retired army physician, refined and gentle, with a keen if fading intellect. I sat one chair away from him and leaned toward him, close, but not too close.

He immediately began his own story of two episodes that occurred after I saw him in the office just a month before: eating dinner at a restaurant, hearing fading away, then, plop, on the floor. Same thing a few days later. I did a quick neurologic review of systems: no aphasia or dysarthria, no weakness, no numbness or diplopia. Simple syncope. Stokes-Adams. Pacer malfunction. Still he talked, needing me to know the details, more than once, of his experience. He was 85, alone, and falling down. I listened. Then the door opened, "Doctor?"

My heart beat faster as I passed through the inner door. I was there to reveal myself, to tell my tale of suffering, and I was embarrassed. Immediately upon entering, I looked up to see my doctor's face. She shot me a look of subtle chagrin, a shared confidence. "This way, Doctor." I sat and waited alone in the examining room for just a moment, heart still beating with anticipation. She came to me immediately. She knew the reason for my visit. My daughters had contracted head lice, and I had been doing battle with them for weeks. The lone adult in my household, I had no one to check me for the loathsome pests and, of course, my head itched constantly. I was mortified at having to seek her help with this problem. That I needed her for this intimate task made me keenly aware of my isolation. She spared me further history taking. She touched my head with sure, gloved hands, beginning the examination without delay, all amid a stream of confidences about how this happened to her once and how awful it was. My doctor's touch, her steady hands, her unmeasured understanding filled me with gratitude and relief. She completed her exam. "Nothing. You are fine."

The business at hand disposed of, she crossed the small room and sat informally on the examination table. (Now let's talk like colleagues. You really are OK, this said to me.) And suddenly it was clear to me that I was not OK. Slowly, I began to tell the real story, not the pretext or the first level of concern. I was sad, very sad. I was struggling at work. I was alone and heartbroken, having just ended an important relationship. There was no one to help me. My children and my patients needed me to be full and overflowing. Instead, I was a well gone dry.

The time allotted for our interview had long since passed. Still this good person, this kind and wise person, looked at me and listened. I felt like a fallen autumn leaf. My voice seemed far away and thin, quite empty of meaning. Still she regarded me. Still she listened and prodded me for more. She saw me clearly, more clearly than I saw myself, and then she very gently told me something painful to hear: "Deb, I think you're depressed." It embarrassed me. I felt exposed and weak. My competence was in question. I recoiled at first, but somehow the courage she showed was like the reach of a firm hand. I took it and was grateful.

The door opened and a nurse poked her head in apologetically. "The architect needs to see this room for renovations." My doctor looked up and said with an edge, "He'll have to wait." Again she turned to me, intent on completing our time together, putting the finishing touches on the creation. "He'll have to wait." I was amazed. Do my patients feel this flood of relief and gratitude? Are my patients healed by kindness in this way? We talked about treatment and I agreed to it "for the children." She refused this self-abrogation. "That doesn't make any sense," she said. "You don't deserve to suffer like this." At the time, I didn't believe her.

We finished, and it was time to leave. As we walked to the waiting room, the nurse mentioned again that the architect had waited for us. "That's the way the cookie crumbles," said my doctor. At that moment, she was a wall for me against the crush of life, a stronghold and safe haven. I was awash in gratitude. My business finished, I returned at last to the waiting room. My patient was not there. I felt alone briefly, but the subtlety of the place reassured me, and I gathered myself to face the day.

Outside was a gloomy March morning. The pewter clouds hung oppressively low. Their cold breath penetrated me, but I made no attempt to secure my jacket. I set out across the parking lot toward the hospital, my heart growing steadily lighter. As I walked, a rich collage of understanding began to dawn on me. Something had just happened. I had been blind. Now my eyes were opened. I had been deaf, and now I could hear. I, the doctor, had been struck low by my human frailty, subject to the same feelings of loneliness, isolation, and overwhelming responsibility that belong to other parents, teachers, professionals. I, the doctor, had experienced the great vulnerability of the patient. I needed help badly, so badly that I did not know how to ask for it. Had my doctor brushed me off or quickly written a prescription, I would have come away injured, not healed. I, the doctor, saw with new eyes my huge power as healer, power that wounds if it is not wielded with compassion. At yet another level, I recognized that what had happened in that examination room was simply an act of love. Love in any relationship, including that between doctor and patient, requires the courage to risk revealing oneself unedited, the willingness to notice and to listen, the willingness to surrender one's own ease or comfort, the willingness to share the suffering of another and the courage to risk and accept gentle confrontation. In this way, any loving relationship can heal. Any relationship hoping to heal without love falls short.

That day, I learned what it is to be in need and be taken care of. That day, I felt healing hands upon me and was left breathless with new awareness of the awesome gift and profound responsibility I had been given as a physician.

River Wind

D. A. FEINFELD, MD

In memory of Dr. Glenda Garvey

Wind off the Hudson slices across
the narrow square by the hospital,
finds bodies and trees, fangs them
with the skill of a mountain cat.
Doctors walk quickly in the street—
a healer's white coat is no shield
to fend off the ravening air.
Safe behind the hospital's brown bricks,
they talk pressure and pulse,
joke about the brain's crazy trails,
rust on the gray goddess's shears.

Amid the sensors' whistles and chirps
that mark heartbeat and breath
Glenda spread her hands
over the sick, out of the wind's way.
Apprentices jostled to be near,

hear her speak, learn the spells
that drive off fever and grief.

Then one day she ran, her black hair
streaming behind, and felt pain
bite through belly and breast.
She knew the track, sure as she knew
branching nerve and vein.
Of course she fought, welcomed inside her
the sting of needle and tube,
like Sebastian taking arrow-points.

Then the tooth-marks slipped
through her like a light gust
between tide-worn sand hills,
left purple scars laid over white
as she thinned to a whirl of cloud.
At the end the storm carried off
her steady voice, her guide,
and she flew off in one final gale,
left the young to remember and grieve.

A healer's white coat is no shield
to fend off the ravening air.

Reflections on a Bone Marrow Transplant

MICHAEL C. DOHAN, MD

I am 63 years old and have been living with chronic lymphocytic leukemia for more than 7 years. Two years ago, progression of symptoms and a worsening hematologic profile despite chemotherapy forced me to make an important personal decision regarding whether or not to receive a bone marrow transplant. As a physician, I knew that transplants for chronic lymphocytic leukemia were controversial and not based on rigorous, controlled studies. It would be risky and difficult, but there was still so much I wanted to do, including living long enough to play an important role in my grandchildren's lives. I chose to go ahead.

After 10 months of chemotherapy, my response was good enough for me to qualify for an autologous transplant. At first I rejoiced, but joy was replaced by anxiety and doubt. Many of those around me—including my physicians, friends, and family—assumed that I, as a physician, had more insight into the proposed therapy than I actually did, heightening the isolation of my decision.

In December 1998, I was admitted overnight for the bone marrow harvest, and the following day I was readmitted to the transplantation service. My room was small and had a special air lock to prevent hospital-borne infections. My wife and any other visitors had to wash and put on a mask and gloves to enter the room. I could leave the room and wander in a tiny hallway only if I put on a mask and gloves. At first, I did not realize how physically and emotionally isolating this space would become.

My therapy started immediately with a double-lumen Hickman catheter. Many of the staff addressed me as "Doctor," which made me feel special. Initially, I played the role by checking the doses of medications, but quickly I found playing doctor-patient to be a struggle. As much as my professional life in medicine had been about control, I needed to let go and trust someone else to care for me. I remembered an editorial that Dr. Franz Ingelfinger had written in the *New England Journal of Medicine* many years ago about his battle with cancer, relating how difficult it was to stop being a consultant in his own case, and how much inner peace he achieved when he finally found a doctor he could trust to treat him as a patient. I needed to do that, too.

Radiation therapy started on the third day. I lay on a trampoline with an x-ray machine above and below me. I quickly learned to time the sessions by counting the clicks of the machines. Every five minutes the machines seemed to shut down briefly and then start up again with a whirring sound. There was nothing physically painful about the radiation, but the sessions were just lonely, and the clicking of the machine seemed like the ticking of a bomb. The radiotherapist had assured me that I would receive a lethal dose—as was therapeutically necessary—and so lethality was always very much on my mind during my trips to therapy. I became weaker and more aware of my feelings of isolation and helplessness. I thought about the survivors of Hiroshima and Nagasaki who had no one waiting in the wings to give them bone marrow back. I wondered what might happen if something went wrong with my harvested marrow and there was none to give back. The progressive and extreme physical and mental weakness accompanied by constant nausea left me with a desire to withdraw from the world. I wished at times that I could just say *"Stop! No more therapy!"* But I never said a word to anyone.

As I reflect back, I find my inability to share my terror with anyone an enigma. Admitting my feelings of terror would have made it harder to deny the reality and to remain a dispassionate physician who believed in the science of this therapy. During those days, I just wanted to lie in bed with the blankets over my head and disappear. I did not know how I would survive. But I forced myself to get out of bed and walk every day and, on a few days, even to ride an exercise bicycle. After these adventures, I would nearly collapse from exhaustion. When I looked up at my intravenous lines—two going constantly, with smaller bags awaiting their turn—I couldn't believe that I was at the other end. I thought of the sick patients in the intensive care unit I had cared for so often with multiple lines going. Now I was on the receiving end of this life-sustaining device, and it was frightening. I wondered whether my patients ever had the same reaction, or whether they found the intravenous bags reassuring.

On the day after the last radiation treatment, my team of doctors, along with several nurses and my wife, gathered around me and, in a 20-minute ceremony, infused my previously purged bone marrow. They didn't lose it. Now began the wait for engraftment.

With the intravenous therapy, I urinated constantly, day and night. One night I slept too soundly and was incontinent of urine. Embarrassed, I changed my surgical scrubs and sheets myself and didn't tell the nurse until morning; she assured me that many patients experience this. The radiation therapy caused severe diarrhea and, later on, so too did the antibiotics. On another night I was incontinent of feces; I rang for the nurse, feeling my last bit of dignity slip away.

As my leukocyte count started to climb, I hung onto every day, hoping it might be the day I'd get to go home. As the day of discharge approached, my nausea intensified and I developed dry heaves. My nurse correctly attributed this to anxiety. That tiny room, which at times seemed like a cell, was, along with the support staff, more important to me than I realized.

On returning home, I decided not to talk to anyone about my experience in the hospital. The few times I attempted to talk about it, I cried. I was totally surprised at how intense my reaction was. When the doctor had warned me that I might have trouble sleeping at home, this seemed preposterous, because nearly all I did in the hospital was sleep. But it was true. I couldn't sleep, despite taking a variety of sleeping pills, and the nausea was worse than ever. I suspected that I was suffering from post-traumatic stress disorder and decided that I had to talk about all that I had been through. My wife and I set up an appointment with a psychiatric social worker. The first meeting was difficult; I cried more than I talked. As a child, I had always been fearful of going to the doctor, and perhaps part of my decision to go into medicine was an effort to master that fear. Now all of that was turned upside down. I was no longer the healer but an utterly helpless patient. That night, I had the first decent sleep since coming home.

On reflection, it's hard to understand why my experience was so difficult and why it had such a severe emotional impact on me. Was it simply because I had never been so sick before? Was it the experience of being brought so close to death with a last-minute rescue? Was it the utter helplessness of the situation, both mental and physical? Was it some effect specific to the therapy? Did having a physician's perspective make all of this more difficult? It was probably all these, and more. What I seem to remember now, months later, was my sense of extreme helplessness, and my inability to muster the strength to fight it. Visitors were most helpful by just being there. Conversation was difficult, and there was little I wanted to do, except to occasionally listen to music. Everything was out of my hands. There was nothing I could do to assure a successful outcome, nothing I could do to make myself feel better, nothing I could do to get back into the world. I just had to wait, and hope. As a doctor, I had always taken pride in caring for others, and, even though I might not always succeed in making my patients better, I was the one in charge. I also was accustomed to feeling in charge of my own health, pursuing athletics and a "healthy" lifestyle with vigor. This experience attacked that sense of control so completely that even now, some emotional fragility remains.

Six months after completing therapy, I resumed my practice part time and felt I had rejoined the living. As I returned to my traditional role as physician, I found I had gained new insights into the doctor-patient relationship. My patients welcomed me back and looked to me for support and help. I, in turn, drew comfort from their trust and regained much strength from returning to the role of healer.

Nine months after transplantation, I visited the unit. The haunting memories made it difficult to go back, but I wanted to thank the staff and show them the success their efforts had achieved. I was surprised at how accessible the unit was. When I went home after the transplantation, it had seemed such a long journey, when in reality it was only a few steps from the elevator. It was good to see the staff. I visited with a young woman going through a similar transplantation. Although a rush of emotion returned, it was not as raw, and I felt I could react appropriately as a patient, doctor, and supporter. It was helpful for both of us.

Much has been written about the impersonalization of modern medical care. The trust we place in our caregivers remains an essential component in recovering from illness. My own physician and other providers were with me every step of the way and their support has been enormously important—important enough that I trusted them to kill me, then bring me back to life.

Balancing the Personal and Professional

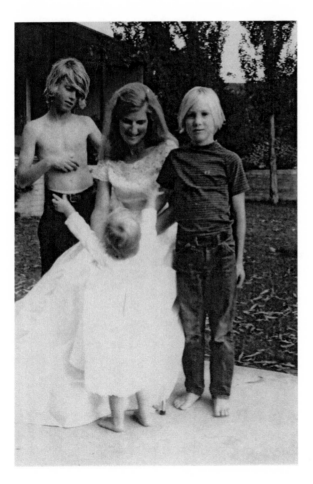

When Did I Know
I Loved Her?

EDWARD V. SPUDIS, MD

Sitting on the U. of Maryland library steps in the sun her
pleated, white tennis dress sent retinal micro-shivers cascading
through my alerted optic chiasm toward asymmetric area-
seventeen sulci, which were then propelled into the nineteens
for, so-called, non-humuncular, dispositional representation—
ignoring mischievous anti-sense oligonucleotide gene noise,
hoping to achieve time-binding(ital) with her flirtatious auditory
parcels being sprayed backward from my naive anterior cinguli,
prompting my immature, unlocalizeable personhood, i.e.,
selfness, to say, "Where's your racket?" fifty years ago.

Untaken Steps and Untold Stories

JOHN D. ROWLETT, MD

I'm not really sure when I first noticed him, proudly sitting on his porch with a broad smile on his weathered face. It was a comforting, peaceful sight—he in his twisted metal chair next to a tattered recliner, greeting the passing world. Most mornings as I hurried down a forgotten hospital access road lined with resident and physician housing, I was blessed with his presence. Countless times I told myself to stop, but I never did. There was always an excuse—a real or perceived crisis, meeting, or event summoning me to the hospital, as if a moth to the light. So, despite his daily proximity, not once during the past seven years did I stop. Not when he was painting his World War II vintage clapboard home a muted yellow. Not when he planted flowers around the porch in spring, picked tomatoes in the summer from the small garden along the road, or raked the leaves from the autumn lawn. And I never stopped on those cool winter mornings when he unbundled his swaddled plants, removing the newspapers that protected them from the erratic Savannah frost. No, I was too busy. I never took the time to share a glass of tea so sweet that it made your pancreas cry, nor did I spend a lazy summer evening breaking butter beans.

My daughter Paige and I never sat in what I am sure was his "guest chair," listening to his stories. I doubt that they were tales of great derring-do or worldly adventures. He, like most of the older persons who made up the neighborhood that envelops this sprawling medical campus, probably traveled little, save for a teenage tour of duty in a distant country or, more recently, for a funeral. Nonetheless, I am sure that there was a purity and richness in his tales. Though I envisioned playing him in checkers, with Paige perched first on my knee and then his, it never happened. I was too busy to hear of the changes in his lifetime or the recalcitrant problems that plague Savannah and the Deep South still. He never reminisced about his grandchildren, though quite possibly some were my patients. No, while I was out doing whatever, he was home. Sitting on his porch, an unspectacular structure supported by cinder blocks, he surveyed his yard as a ruler his kingdom. And I was figuring out my next project while he watched me and the rest of the world drive past. Although the tattered recliner was always unoccupied, he appeared content—satisfied, I think, with a life well lived.

I've been to countless resuscitations over the past two decades. Some were successful, most not. Almost without exception, they were strangers. I've searched secretion-filled throats looking for landmarks and sliding plastic, hopefully, through the instruments of their voice—a voice that told stories to people whom I was yet to meet or might never meet. Inserting catheters and needles into arms that held children, grandchildren, and loved ones with occasional precision but directed purpose. Assaulting them in a last ditch effort to stave off the inevitable. We are mortal. Regardless of intent, success, or professionalism, we are inevitably strangers at a most personal time.

It's July now. For the past two weeks, the quiet access road has been filled with moving vans. First, with those of our graduates, off to "real world" medicine—to battle with insurance companies, hospital administration, medical records, and, oh yes, most importantly, to make a difference. In-Training Examination scores have been wonderful. We have taught them, and they have taught themselves, and each other, well. Each is an excellent clinician. Now, this week, empty boxes appear on the curb, discarded by the new crew, the interns. Eager eyes and accepting minds, waiting to be taught. Waiting to get into the game. Ready to matter. Ready to learn what we teach, both explicit and implicit.

His house is for sale; the sign appeared last week. The chair, his chair, is empty. An immaculate older-model sedan is parked in the front yard. The grass needs mowing. I'd like to believe he moved— maybe to a place where people took the time to talk with him, to play checkers, or just to sit quietly in the tattered recliner. But I doubt it. His generation, that of my parents, tends not to move by choice (particularly when they already live in a warm climate). No, most likely he died. And although I do not know his name or his fate, it is distinctly possible, perhaps probable, that one of our resident physicians held the laryngoscope. Better someone had held his hand. I just hope he, or she, unlike me, stopped long enough to say hello before his good-bye.

Tomorrow I will greet my new intern. He too is eager. He called last week wanting to know what to do on his first day, what he should expect. I wonder what he'll say when I tell him I want to take a walk, drink some tea, and play checkers. I want him to learn about life from those who know it best. And who better from whom to learn than those who have lived it most? And maybe I'll sneak a little medicine in there just for fun.

Northwoods Elegy

DAVID P. STEENSMA, MD

The paddles we grip are aspen and white pine. Our canoe's thwarts are cedar; the heavy yoke of the canoe is varnished maple, carved from the same tall trees that rim this remote northern lake. As our boat glides through thick morning mist, I kneel in the stern and gently steer us away from the ripples that warn of unforgiving boulders just beneath the water's dark surface. Up in the bow, an old friend is scanning the shoreline, hoping to catch sight of a moose.

Although he is a lifelong city dweller, my canoe mate was chosen for this trip because he is gifted with a key backwoods instinct—a keen sense of when to speak up and when to keep quiet. On windless mornings like today, we take pride in echoing the stillness of woods and water as we pull our paddles through the cold depths in total silence. When we carry out this motion perfectly, the lake rewards us with small whorls that spin off into the distance, farther than we can track them.

We have come to the Boundary Waters Canoe Area in northern Minnesota, a chain of a thousand lakes connected by short rocky trails for portaging. Surrounded by iron mines and scattered over a million acres of pristine wilderness hard on the Canadian border, the Boundary Waters exert a magnetic tug on those of us who love the rhythm of the paddle. My companion and I are here for a weeklong respite from the jangling chaos of modern life. I've retreated to the woods often with this end in mind, and each time I leave exhausted but re-freshed—briefly dazzled by the extravagance of electricity and central heating, ready again to face another year of the urgent demands of pagers, papers, and patients.

I've learned from past trips that it may be easy to escape the daily routine of the clinic, but it is not so simple to leave the patients be-hind. Thoughts of people whose stories I have been privileged to hear creep up on me in quiet moments like this. Most are welcome guests, but others—especially those for whom I might have done better—are a burden, more irritating than a heavy canoe digging into my shoul-ders on a long, dusty, late afternoon portage. During breaks from pad-dling, when my friend and I let our small boat drift aimlessly in the current, listening to the water lap gently against the gunwales, I often find myself puzzling over an ongoing difficult case, wondering how an old patient is doing or simply remembering. Today I can't get the French man out of my mind.

I met him the winter after the "Big Blowdown." On Independence Day 1999, a *derecho*—an inland hurricane that doesn't waste any en-ergy spinning—smashed through these northern woods with 90-mile-per-hour winds, twisting thick timber into broken tangles. Trees were felled in a 12-mile-wide strip 30 miles long, rendering huge ar-eas of familiar country unrecognizable.

The Frenchman suffered a crisis of his own that fatal summer. It started as a stitch in his side, an unpredictable jab just under his ribs. After a few weeks, the pain became enough of an annoyance for him to make an appointment to see his doctor for a physical. When his urine turned brown and his skin a waxy yellow, the consultation was ur-gently rescheduled. The usual scans and biopsies were performed, and the black news was cancer—probably a cholangiocarcinoma, maybe something else; the pathologists couldn't really tell, but given the stage it really didn't matter. A biliary stent was inserted. Surgery was not possible; chemotherapy quickly failed.

I saw him at the Mayo Clinic in Rochester for a second opinion during the dreariest part of the midwestern winter. He had reached a stage where it was obvious from the moment I set eyes on him that death was not far away. His canary-colored skin hung in loose folds from wasted limbs, and as he told me the story of his suffering, he looked at me through tired, mustard-tinted eyes. There was nothing that could be done for him beyond arranging to have his stent changed, but he really hadn't expected much from me anyway. He confessed that he had come only because his family insisted on being certain everything possible had been done before they would accept the inevitable. Finally, to keep the peace at home, he allowed his sons to drive him to Rochester to seek out that black seal of incurability that Mayo doctors are often called upon to provide.

With nothing for me to recommend, we spent our allotted time talking about his life in the north and trading stories about favorite lakes in the Boundary Waters. Although his surname was French and his parents had once lived on the edge of the Iron Range, he did not know if he had come from Voyageur stock. Still, his passions were canoeing and fishing, and he had once been a passable deer hunter, so he joked that if he actually were descended from those hardy fur traders, they would not be disappointed in him. As soon as his young sons could hold a rod, he had taught them how to icefish; now that they were grown men with families and ice sheds of their own, routinely hauling in more walleye, pike, and lake trout than he had ever done himself, he felt that he had done his duty and accepted that his life would soon end. When our conversation finally ebbed, we shook hands. I noted that despite his wasted arms, his grip was strong— probably still muscular enough to handle a paddle.

All the following summer, as the Forest Service anxiously watched the injured Boundary Waters for the wildfires that start so easily in downed timber, the French man's liver filled with metastatic embers from his own internal blaze. I later learned that he had lasted longer than anyone who saw him the previous winter might have guessed— at least if they had not felt his firm grasp as I had. But by the time I took to the woods again myself the following September, he was gone.

The northern wilderness is exhilarating in early fall. The days are not yet perceptibly shorter, but nights are already sharp with cold. At last night's island campsite, the chill bit deeply into my skin whenever I strayed a few paces from the fireside. I emerged from our tent this morning to find the edges of the lake coated with a rime of ice; we brushed frost off our paddles before setting out. But the reward for our fortitude is solitude. After the school term starts and summer camps close, the number of canoeists dwindles. In mid-September, a carefully chosen route through this wilderness offers the chance to travel for days without seeing another person; in July, it would take a sailplane and a crossing into Canada to make such a bold escape.

As we make camp for the last time, my friend notes excitedly that few mosquitoes and blackflies survived the previous night's hard frost. Soon we are huddled around another fire ring, listening to the plaintive wails of distant loons as the cold evening air slowly encroaches. The night sky, which has stunned us with its clarity all week, is muted tonight—another casualty of the ice. We are ready to go home.

It is not easy to return to the clinic after a time away. The ills that afflict modern medicine seem magnified by distance. With each passing year, I feel a little less like the caring doctor I once envisioned and more like a salmon running upstream, butting up against powerful currents flowing swiftly in the wrong direction. Physicians on the verge of retirement share their sorrow that I chose to enter the profession just at it was getting to be no fun; this does not help. I spend too much of the year wishing I had stayed in the woods.

Still, it remains a special gift to be allowed to stand by patients in their time of need, even when, as with the Frenchman, there is little I can do to relieve their suffering. I may never have the autonomy of my medical forebears; I seem destined to spend more time with paperwork and the output of machines, and I will certainly be less wealthy. But as long as I get to hear the stories of patients and carry them with me wherever I go, even deep into the woods, medicine will not lose its ability to pull me out of the lakes.

Double Helix

ANGELEE DEODHAR

Now a housewife, once a surgeon
a template for the DNA chain
like the double helix of her being
she's reduced to wearing latex gloves
only while housecleaning every week
meticulously she dons cap, mask, apron

on a trolley arranged with surgical precision
lie her gloves, brushes, dusters, solutions
she drapes furnitures with sheets of cotton
then pulls on her gloves tightens them
her size a neat seven

she prepares the area to be cleaned
with a weak Savlon solution
swabs it as she would an abdomen
in precise deft strokes
from above below left to right
never using an extra movement

and just as she had once done in the OR
she keeps soft music on—Strauss, Vivaldi
she wonders if now her DNA double helix
carries two genes
one for housewife one for surgeon

squeeze-drying the mop each time
she scrubs the floor surgically clean
removes the trolley
absently counting her instruments
removes gloves, cap, mask, apron
the overshoes

washes off the excess powder
from her hands and creams them
looking at them critically thrombosed
blue-veined yet soft supple
she warms them with her mug of coffee
and then takes up her pen
to write a poem.

Glass Ceiling

BHUVANA CHANDRA, MD

Almost, it seemed, I smelled
the patch of withered grass, the green of stale,
imbued with glutinous spit, now dried;
as integral a part of his scuffed leather shoe soles
as orange bug-splatters on a windshield.
My nostrils curled. He shifted
so his right shoe angled on the glass topped desk
and the left pointed, like a sword, at my shoulder,
its steel tip awash in smug aplomb.
From my seat, my vision framed
by his shod legs, modern caveman clubs,
I watched the metronome
of his breath, up, down, up, down,
stirring the point of his purple striped tie
on his polyester covered abdominal dune.
I thought of my great-aunt,
the one who did not turn up
at her own wedding, an arranged marriage.
"I'm not chattel," she said, and insisted

on an apology from the groom she dumped.
My interviewer stretched back in his swivel chair
and clasped his hands behind his hunter head.
"I hope you don't plan on getting pregnant,
we have problems with calls then, you know.
The men sure have it hard."
His feet remained lollygagging, eye-to-eye with me.
All I could think of was the story of my grandmother,
about how she died after the birth of my father
with a weak smile of apology,
as if she had failed her husband
with all that hemorrhaging.
"Well," he straightened up at last,
brought his feet back to floor with a thud.
"You've got the job." Jots of loosed dirt
shimmied on the glass.
I hoped he took off his shoes
before his next appointment, scrubbed them hard,
for if not
he would always stink
of saliva, chewed gum, crushed weeds and inferiority.

Magic in the Web of It

LORI A. BORELLA, MD

We give up a lot to do this job. Medicine's a vocation, really. Calling it a job doesn't address the sacrifices we make. How often do we miss meals, miss sleep, or miss our families for patients? Sometimes our dedication to medicine causes us to lose our families entirely. Why, then, do we do it? We do it because medicine gives us something in return. Occasionally, that something is extraordinary. That something happened to me.

In the fall of my third year of medical school, I had the opportunity to do a rural medicine clerkship in Valentine, Nebraska, a small ranching community in the northwest corner of the state. Students who had previously worked with the doctors in Valentine each had a story to tell—everything from manic tourists to farmers kicked by a surly bovine. What would my story be?

After one week in Valentine, I had no stories to tell. The days were relatively mundane conglomerations of managing hypertension and performing well-child checks. Doldrums in medicine are often short lived. A lunchroom conversation with a medical technician ended mine.

"You know, Lori, you really remind me of a nurse who used to work here."

"So, you have a lot of gorgeous, brilliant blondes here in Valentine, huh?" I jokingly replied.

I didn't give the conversation a second thought. However, the following week her comment was echoed by the physicians, phlebotomists, and pharmacists. Half the staff was engaged in casual banter about my "carbon copy." Whoever this nurse was, I walked like her, talked like her, laughed like her, and wrinkled my nose like her. I had a twin, or so it seemed.

As luck would have it, my "twin" was scheduled to come into the clinic the following week. Finally, a chance to see the remarkable resemblance everyone was talking about. Unfortunately, I never got the chance to meet her. During her appointment, I was dealing with another patient's gouty toe and saw just the back of her head as she walked out the clinic door. Like all jokes, this one had an expiration date. No more quips about my doppelgänger were made in the days that followed.

Five days later, I scrubbed in on a melanoma excision. While the surgeon closed, the scrub nurse, anesthetist, and I made conversation. The scrub nurse said to me, "Have you lived in Rapid City your whole life?"

I replied, "Almost; I was in a foster home for three months before I was adopted."

Forceps clattered to the floor. Silence. The anesthetist's eyes were bigger than God's ego. I imagined the scrub nurse's mouth dropping open behind her surgical mask. She spoke again: "You aren't going to believe this ... I can't believe this!"

"Believe what?" I asked.

She hesitated. "This woman ... this woman you look exactly like gave up a baby for adoption."

She was right—I wasn't going to believe it. I was offended that she would take a joke to that extent. I then realized she wasn't laughing. When the levee of shock gave way, my tears threatened to break the sterile field. I maintained some semblance of control until the last knot was tied. After the procedure, the scrub nurse approached me in the locker room. She had gone to high school with this woman and had pictures of her. Did I want to see them?

The following evening, I went to the scrub nurse's house and drank a soda that I did not taste, while she rifled through her dusty annuals. She flipped past fading penned sentiments of "Friends 4 Ever" and stopped on a photo of a teenage girl. I could not breathe. I could not blink. It was my face. I was suddenly looking at my own high school yearbook. My mind was paralyzed by sheer disbelief, but in my heart, I knew—this woman had to be my birth mother.

What now? A collision of nature and nurture? Do I even want this? What if she's a bad person? Do our hands look the same? Would she be proud of me? Has she ever regretted her decision to give me up? The resolution of my fears and answers to the questions about where I came from and who I am was only a few miles away on a Nebraska cattle ranch. The Fates had taken my hand to this point. Could I go the distance?

I called her on a Thursday evening. Was this the beginning or end of my story?

We met four days later.

The Other Résumé

MICHAEL A. COTTON, MD

Clearing away the kids' educational CDs from my desktop, I settled down in front of the computer. Well into my second year of residency in internal medicine, I figured it was time to update my résumé. Just a month before, my wife and I had struggled with the question of whether I should pursue a fellowship in critical care. I had obtained an application and even filled it out, but family considerations supervened. We both agreed that it would be better to leave training behind and begin my career rather than to prolong our current lifestyle with yet another educational segue.

Outside my window, newly fallen snow sparkled in the sunshine of a crisp winter day. Opening my word processing file, I started the laborious task. First section: education. I had done well in medical school, generally excelling and receiving several honors along the way. Residency, however, had been different. The kids were continuing to grow older and their demands of me were greater. When I wasn't sleeping, my time was theirs, not mine. The extra polish that I had been able to produce in medical school was no longer there. Would more reading at night or on the weekends have made a difference on rounds or in morning report? Maybe I would have been more confident, more insightful, more impressive. Maybe I could have been a chief resident... .

Next came the topic of licensure. I had passed Step III during internship, thus earning the right to a state medical license. In another 18 months, I would be eligible to take the internal medicine boards. Each step in the testing process had witnessed a decrease in my performance compared to that of my peers, with a recent in-training exam seeming to confirm that even more of my fellow residents were better prepared for the practice of medicine than I. Once again, the unwelcome questions intruded: Not enough time studying? Not enough dedication? Not enough knowledge to give the best care to my patients?

I skipped the next logical section, publications, because it was empty. No, it was hollow. I like to teach and at times had wondered about academics; now, that thought seemed like a foolish fancy. Without papers or posters, could I seriously pursue a faculty position? Medical students with whom I worked had frequently expressed appreciation for my teaching, but I had never been published. Besides, did I know enough to be a good teacher?

Finally: employment. Here I had a little meat. After graduating from college and marrying, I worked for four years while my wife finished her elementary education degree. The job wasn't always exciting, but I learned from the work world an endurance that I hadn't learned as a student. For the next three years, I did various things, intermingling international travel with seminary coursework before returning to work and applying to medical school. Surely, that time counted for something, even if only to me ... and my wife. During those seven years, before the challenges and strains of medical school and residency, we solidified our marriage and created a strong home for the children God would give us.

My reverie was interrupted as my 3-year-old daughter and 6-year-old son burst into the office, pleading me to join them in the snow. Acquiescing, I put on my boots and coat and trudged outside. Surely, I thought, these are the things that have altered the balance, making my résumé less than I had hoped it would be.

Braced by the chill, dazed by the sunlight, I crunched through the snow, playing chase and preparing snowballs for a real cold war. Soon I was infected with my kids' boundless excitement. My wife, pregnant with our third, joined us, and we all had the time of our lives. The computer seemed far away. Yes, I was a doctor, but I was a husband and a father. Maybe my professional record was not all that I might have wished, but, thank God, I had another résumé.

Obstetricians Wanted:
No Mothers Need Apply

LAUREN PLANTE, MD

I was an obstetrician, and then I was a mother, until I had to give up the one for the other.

This wasn't the way I planned it, and I grieve for the loss. I spent four years in medical school and another eight in residency, and I always assumed I would work until I dropped. I wasn't dissuaded by the length of training, or the $100,000 worth of loans, or the inroads on my nights and weekends. No, I envisioned a career filled with satisfying clinical work, grateful patients, and ongoing intellectual challenges, in which I would always rise to the occasion. In a parenthetical kind of way, I knew some people who began families in medical school, and some in residency; there were even a few brave souls who had children before they were in medical school. What choices they had to make, I don't know; I wonder now, but it didn't register then.

During the time I was in training, obstetrics and gynecology became, in more ways than one, a women's specialty. I vividly remember one obstetrics–gynecology department chairman, incensed because several of his chief residents were pregnant, harrumphing that there was no place for pregnant women in his specialty. That was before women made up, as they do today, the majority of residents in the field. There has, in fact, been concern expressed that it's difficult now for young male obstetrician–gynecologists to find work because so many women prefer to see a female gynecologist. Women have flocked to this field in the belief that we have something of value to offer, and many patients seem to agree. Perhaps it's shared experience, or, to borrow a phrase, the view from the other end of the speculum.

Although we take care of women, we don't take care of our women. When, at age 37, I delivered my firstborn one week to the day after beginning a fellowship in high-risk pregnancy, I was devastated to have him admitted to the neonatal intensive care unit. On my way out the door, I ran into the senior fellow, who said to me, "Too bad about what happened. When can I put you back on the call schedule?" I seriously considered skipping my four allotted weeks of maternity leave, since if both my son and I were at the hospital, I could arrange to see him more. Little has changed since then: Our residents get a few weeks off for maternity leave, after which they must either resume their 12-hour days (and every third or fourth night in the hospital) or add extra time to their four years of residency training. Personally, I think that any obstetrics–gynecology trainee who dares to have a baby during her residency is entitled to extra credit: elective time, perhaps. When I made this suggestion in the pages of *Obstetrics & Gynecology*, it provoked outrage.

Obstetrics is a 24-hour, 7-day-a-week specialty. The pattern used to be that a new physician worked mostly in obstetrics, and as he aged along with his patients (and got tired of being up all night), he stopped delivering babies and switched over to gynecology. It's hard to predict what will happen now that the face of the specialty is less male. A woman who has children quickly realizes that they, too, are a 24-hour, 7-day-a-week specialty. A woman who put off having any children until she finished training finds that starting a practice and a family simultaneously leaves her always wondering where she falls short. A woman who waits until her practice is established winds up staring down her biological clock. The infertility specialist is up against the same constraints as her patients.

Creative options are few. The recent escalation in the cost of malpractice insurance coverage has largely precluded options for part-time practice; the physician who delivers one patient per month pays just as high a rate as everyone else. At my academic medical center, premiums in my department increased by 68% last year, which brought the base rate to $100,000 per physician per year. (Some of my colleagues were assessed twice that.) A number of senior men, but interestingly enough, none of the women, promptly gave up obstetrics altogether and switched to a predominantly surgical gynecology practice. When I asked to cut back to a 4-day work week, I was told I couldn't possibly generate enough revenue to cover the expense of keeping me, what with salary, overhead, and liability insurance.

Babies bloomed in my department in the year 2000: Two obstetrics–gynecology faculty members and three residents gave birth to children. One was a first-time mother, and four had done it before and had somehow made it work. Now, a couple of years later, so many of our solutions have proved impermanent. One is still practicing, but the other four could not reconcile the competing demands, nor add more hours to the day. Most mornings, I'd leave my sleeping children with my kisses cooling on their cheeks, and then I'd see them for an hour or two in the evenings—just enough time to fight over homework, dinner, and bedtime, assuming I wasn't on the phone with a patient or on my way back to the hospital. I believe—I hope—my patients will miss me, but I am certain my children did.

These constraints are not specific to the specialty. Women in many fields of medicine, or for that matter in many professions, labor under the same burdens. But in obstetrics and gynecology, we talk a great deal about respecting choices women make, which means we might discuss the pros and cons of hormone replacement therapy or whether to deliver by cesarean. If we gave more than lip service to the importance of women's choices, we would recognize how unpalatable are the choices we leave ourselves; we would question the paradigm that imposes the necessity for such choices. We would strive to find creative solutions, whether that means flex-time, shared time, team care with nonphysician providers, in-hospital child care, or a hospitalist model with shifts on the labor floor. We would be willing to experiment, even willing to fail, because the system as it now stands is failing us.

We would advocate for a system that enables women to have both children and a satisfying professional life, whether those women are our patients, our colleagues, or ourselves.

The Middle Time

MICHAEL AYLWARD, MD

The people on the road just do not understand the need to drive a little faster, to brake a little less, and, generally, to get out of my way. Frustration and resentment are not too far under my skin after 30-odd hours of wakefulness and decision making.

I barrel around a circular on-ramp that straightens out and immediately splits into three highways. I curse the confusing design as I drive by a single-file line of traffic to my right. Sheep, I think, they are all sheep, lining up good and early to keep me from getting home, getting to bed. I cut into the line just before the exit—a New York move that I never performed until moving to Minnesota. Everyone else is coming home from a day's work—I've got two days under my belt, doesn't that give me some kind of priority? Well, it should.

The light three blocks from my apartment marks the beginning of the worst part of the trip. The light itself is usually fairly short. I zip across Lagoon, past the grocery store parking lot on the left. That last word—left—is the bane of my post-call existence. Minnesotans cannot turn left without much braking, contemplation, hemming, and sloth. I slide past the left-turners, swerve back in front of them (narrowly avoiding the parked car), and gas it to the next light, where, usually, the walk signal is blinking. Occasionally, a yellow light is run.

Sometimes, I don't make the light. So I wait, angry at the world for the redness of the light, the slowness of the cars, my smell, and the 4:00 A.M. chronic obstructive pulmonary disease admission. Eventually, the light turns green, and I go.

My memory is short when I am tired—the small slights of the night before and the drive home slip out of my thoughts as I turn onto my street. I am calm by the time I pull in front of my apartment and walk directly into the shower.

I molt. A layer of grime and sweat slides off along with the anxiety of the previous night and with the frustration of the pager and those on the other end of it. I take my wad of clothes and throw them, en bloc, into the hamper. There is no sneaking one more wear out of these.

I lie down on my blue corduroy recliner, sit back, and put something, anything, on the TV. Finally, the puppeteers strings are snipped, and I slip without conscience into the deepest blackness I know—a dreamless, instantaneous passage of time. I am in a relativistic vessel, reaching the speed of light briefly as the world goes by ... .

Sometimes, I wake up and do not know where I am or what time it is. My wife says words, but they make no sense. I reply, and I don't make any sense. It's nonsense. My eyes barely see. I. Just. Want. To. Sleep.

Sometimes, I wake rested, ready to spend a few hours being productive or lazy or creative. Making dinner, doing laundry.

Sometimes I wake, and it is the next day.

By morning, I am back—a thinking person once again, no longer one of Dostoyevsky's "men of action." The tension in my shoulders is gone, and I am in balance once again. I glide through the morning easily, without weight. My pager is lighter as I clip it onto my belt on the way to the car.

The clarity of the next day is almost worth the fog of the previous one. I notice it most on my walk from the parking garage to the hospital. My steps are crisp, my mind clear. The sky is bluer, the grass is greener, and the red bricks of the hospital are rough and cool. The grout between the bricks crumbles under my fingertips without touching it. I smell sap oozing out of the trees. The world is not flat on the walk to work. There is depth.

By the time the hospital swallows me up and I re-enter the short call, pre-call, call, post-call cycle, I am re-focused. It is really not about me, after all. My patients are waiting, and they never went home.

Our Medical Marriage

RICHARD M. BERLIN, MD

for Susanne

We kneeled on the bookstore floor
two students scanning the bodies
of new books, checking out
each other's *Principles*
of Internal Medicine.
Scores of textbooks later
we're a pair of pagers and missed dinners,
companions in sleep-deprived nights.
We suffered the long delay
before our only child while we ran
to slashed wrists and ODs,
sprinted from half-read journal
to school play to board meeting.
In conversation long as summer light
we talked patients and drugs,
recited the crushed prayers of the dying,

learned how we both took medicine
as a life-long lover.

One hushed June evening in mid-life
scented rose and thick with fireflies,
the phone steals her.
I sit with my unfilled glass
and a life we knew we were choosing,
our marriage a joining of two strains
of mint, planted close, cross-pollinated
to form a single type, the small, unfailing
flowers arrayed in purple spikes
I can see most clearly
when I'm down on my knees.

A Walk on the Beach

ANTHONY JOSEPH CHIARAMIDA, MD

The wind invites me, tired, out to the sandy beach
It stretches out before me, endless beneath my feet.
Warm, and soft, and yielding,
A bed for me to sleep.

And as I bend down slowly,
A smile on my face,
I try to grab some handfuls
But the grains, too small, don't stay.

And they slide between my fingertips,
Despite the tighter grip
And I smile again to realize
That the sand remains in place.

For others who will come,
Tired of their fates,
And rest their souls upon the breast
And warm heart of this beach.

So I walk up to the water,
And listen to the waves,
As they offer conversation
Filled with freshness, a delight.

Again I bend down slowly,
A smile on my face
And I try to grab some handfuls
But the drops, too small, don't stay.

And they slip between my fingertips,
Despite my tighter grip
And I smile again to realize
That the waves remain in place.

For others who will come,
Tired of their fates,
And rest their souls upon the breast
And warm heart of this beach.

So I walk down past the breakers,
My face against the wind
And listen to the whispers
Spin a welcome voice of peace.

I bend down once more, slowly,
A smile on my face,
And I try to grab some handfuls
But the winds, too quick, don't stay.

And they slide between my fingertips,
Despite the tighter grip
And I smile again to realize
That the wind remains in place.

For others who will come,
Tired of their fates,
And rest their souls upon the breast
And warm heart of this beach.

And I laugh unto myself
As have the waves and sand and wind,
To think to take away the parts
That make this place a whole.

And I thank them one more time,
As I turn to say goodbye.
Again they fill my heart with love
And my soul they fill with joy.

And what I take I cannot hold,
And I leave what stays with me,
And I await the time again,
When my friend will meet with me.

Blue Light and Milk

DAVID A. MOROWITZ, MD

While it doesn't seem important now that I can't remember the exact date or even the month it happened, it seems significant that I was nearing the end of a medical fellowship and that the weather then was clear and cold. And since my son was about 5 months old, the special night related here must have been in early winter, perhaps January. Yet while his age and the time of year are related to the quality and simple events of that night, it is what I learned about filial love and fatherhood that remains so precise and crisp in my memory. And it was a long time ago. That little boy is now 30 years old, my age when this all happened, and, at 60, I have since doubled the years of my life. The symmetry in our age changes certainly enhances the recollection.

This near-magical adventure began at about 3:00 A.M., when I was awakened by my infant son's crying. So that he wouldn't disturb my wife or our 2-year-old daughter, I quickly left my warm bed for the cooler air of our apartment and the sad baby's side. His frustrated, inarticulate tears were traced to a chilled, wet diaper and a presumption of hunger. Lifting him out of his crib, I rested his sobbing little body on the left side of my chest and, with his moistened diaper and buttocks secure on my forearm, plopped barefoot on uncarpeted floors into the kitchen. With the dexterity of early adulthood, I was able to open our refrigerator door with my right hand, find one of the already prepared and waiting bottles of milk and infant formula, locate a saucepan and partially fill it with water, ignite the jets on the gas stove, and set the pan and an upright bottle to warming. Our journey continued into the bathroom where, with a shut door protecting my wife's sleep, I turned on the light; removed my son's cold, yellowed, and weighty clothing; and, holding him safely in our sink, gave his underside its much-needed soapy, tepid bath. Then, with the crying done and old tears disappearing, he was placed, dry and powdered, into a new diaper, hearing reassurances about his bigness, his goodness, and the love his parents and sister bore him.

Tired father and hungry son then repeated the trip to the kitchen, the bottle by now acceptably warm, and retired to his bedroom for an early morning feeding. Our home was on the fourth floor of a large, U-shaped university-owned building. We lived at its deep concave center, from which the two parallel arms reached forward toward a quiet street, a vacant schoolyard, and, over both that clear winter night, a perfect full moon whose reflected luminance filled a cloudless sky and this little boy's bedroom with a deep, sapphire-blue light. I sat at the foot of a single bed adjacent to his crib, rested his shoulders in the fold of my left arm and his buttocks on my thigh, and inserted the milky nipple into his expectant mouth. Strong little muscles began their exuberant work, my right wrist rhythmically pulled in and thrust out as he struggled impatiently to empty the bottle's load and satisfy his hunger.

Imagine, then, what I recall so easily: a dark room, filled by an even, blue radiance, outlining the furniture and us. The only sounds were of his sucking and our dissimilar breathing, mine growing progressively slower. Within minutes, as a consequence of my "on-call" schedule, I began to doze, dropping my lids down for 1, then 2, and then perhaps 3 or more seconds. As I tipped slowly forward, my internal sensors shook me awake to see a baby's eyes fixed on my face. They were unblinking, widely opened, whites fully exposed, seeming to grasp at my image as avidly as he was devouring that bottle. To him that early morning, I could have had no name or title, but this certainly was one moment when his mind linked my face to the pleasure of feeding, to warm arms that kept him from falling, to the relief of cold wetness, and to hands that were washer, dryer, and powderer of flesh. We sat there, loving parent and attentive, wordless child, young father and younger son, mutually enchanted, I hypnotized by the vision of his bright new eyes searching my face, pulling who knows how many signals about me into that acquisitive, unfettered intelligence.

But the learning was not all his. Amidst the acrobatics of bath, food, security, and warmth, that clear blue night whispered how absolutely our lives were being joined. Though still cocooned within his soft, sweet-smelling skin, his quickly filling brain, and his poorly controlled musculature, our embraces foreshadowed the anticipated pleasures of shared softball games, meals, and bedtimes, but also the sacrifices he would endure because of my life as a physician. I could also grasp a momentary glimmer of his fatherhood; his tiny body, like my larger one, surely would be the first conduit of another life, equally dependent on him, conceived in love and joined, as mine was to his, by a different kind of love.

This was our night, a man's night. His sister and mother, my daughter and wife, both uninvolved, remained asleep and unaware. Eventually, though, I was overcome by fatigue. I trudged back to the kitchen with my drowsy child and rinsed out bottles. Then we returned, in proper sequence, to our different dreams.

This unforgettable night occurred when his education as a human seemed to begin and my formal academic training was ending. We have since moved from that apartment and that city, managed to survive my own father's death, and, despite the intrusions of my medical work, prospered as a family. Yet, as he begins and I end our second thirty years living hundreds of miles apart, a change I could not have foreseen has taken place. His needs have been replaced by my own, an increasing desire for his company. Using a curiosity about his work, colleagues, and social life as an excuse, I call him regularly, sometimes daily. Disregarding my likely intrusiveness and the too-modest guilt in keeping my patients waiting a bit longer, I punch his number on my desk telephone, first hearing his receptionist's knowing, respectful greeting, then relegated to my place "on hold." It is my chance to reflect, the nuisance's penitence: Do I rely on his courtesy as he once did my fatherly obligations? Does he resent my selfish interruptions? Then I also wonder if, between our calls, he and his sister have those understandable, young adult thoughts about parents: their ever-swidening middles, embarrassing repetitive anecdotes, failing hearing, and certainly that occasional flash about when or how "it" will happen. But the considerate, cheery, "Hi, Pop!" rescues me, and we're together again, bonded as always. Did I forget, even briefly, that he loves me too?

Sixty; thirty; one. While most episodes of early fatherhood are forgotten and that part of our time together was predictable, the feelings still overwhelm. I marvel at how much of me is in him: our mutual tastes and dislikes, the nearly identical cadences of our footfalls, the times when old friends cannot distinguish our voices. I can't explain this except in the vaguest biological or emotional terms. But feeling the warmth of his voice or his broad, reassuring man's hand on my shoulder, I travel by reflex back half my lifetime and nearly all of his, returning in thought to a night when his eyes wouldn't leave my face, when the links of love and comfort were forged in the resolute watchfulness of a father by his infant son, a nocturne of blue light and milk, the mysterious beginnings of love.

Those Who Are
Our Patients

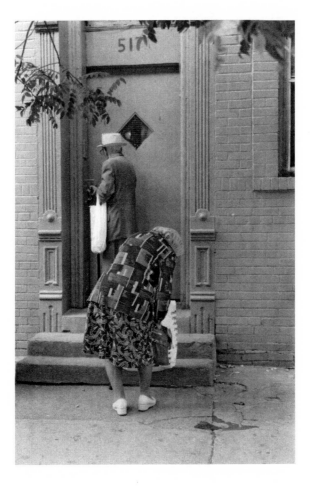

Haven

TIMOTHY LAHEY, MD

I drive in,
pelted by hail.
Each impact feels like a curse,
a bitter recollection
of our minor atrocities,
our inability to be concerned.
After I park, and run,
my white coat gets wet,
and weighs heavier by the second.
Entering, I await the moment that
the beeping and whirring inside,
disguise the staccato rebuke
of the storm outside.

For even the way
you placed in the palm of the wife's hand
the spider,
the bitter news of her husband's demise,
was a blessing.
You allowed that

his very last weeks with a tube in his trachea,
his nightmarish swim in rocket fuel and haze,
were ultimately an insult to inevitability,
the ravaging coccus.
You were there not to look away;
you delivered her to her time of deepest bewilderment,
and eventually, gently, abandoned her there.

In the next chamber,
the brusque ICU nurse cries,
seeing her patient obtain that imperceptible chance
of life again,
his once inhuman and edematous arm
lifting dance-like from the bed,
reaching and unmistakably vital.
This is my haven here,
where for all the ugly denial
of daylight's name,
moments of undiluted good arrive
unexpectedly, mercilessly,
like an undeserved benediction,
and behind the thick windows,
the world rages, unheard.

Trust

SAMUEL C. DURSO, MD

"How'd you miss that frog, Doc?" There was a tinge of irritation in Ezra's voice.

No use making an excuse. I steadied my balance, planting both feet astride the flat-bottomed boat and squeezed my eyes shut to stop the stinging. Sweat ran over my brow, down my cheeks and into the corners of my mouth. It had a bitter, coppery taste from the headlamp.

"That's awright. Don't worry about it. I'll put you on another one."

Ezra could be a demanding teacher, but he was also practical. Razzing me wasn't going to put more frogs in the boat. There were half a dozen in a burlap bag behind me. In spite of countless forays hunting and fishing together in the marsh, frogging was new to me.

I opened my eyes and replanted my feet in anticipation of our moving. He eased his paddle over the side of the boat and pushed us forward out of the thick algae and grass.

"Let's go over there. Should be some frogs in those lily pads, Doc."

A click followed by the soft electric purr of the trolling motor, and Ezra maneuvered us into open water. The din of insect sounds subsided as our movement created a little artificial breeze. By then I had stopped thinking about the mosquitoes. I stood over the front of the boat holding a 10-foot pole tipped with a spring-action gig, concentrating on keeping my balance and looking for the reflection of frog eyes in my headlight.

The nighttime marsh was alternately black and silver. Overhead, little patches of spring sky shone, and occasionally the moon could be seen peeping through heavy clouds. It might rain. My headlight swept ahead 20 or 30 feet. I looked over the side of the boat and let my lamp beam penetrate the tea-colored water. Except for a brown-green glow, I saw nothing.

"Keep your head inside the boat, Doc. We run over an alligator and startle it, it could lash its tail gittin' outta the way an' take your head off. I seen a guy get his neck broke that way."

Something to remember. I redirected my light beam ahead of the boat looking for the white reflection of frog eyes. Snake and turtle eyes were different. I looked out for alligator eyes too.

I was struck by the irony of this doctor–patient relationship. In the office our relationship was somewhat conventional; he was deferential and treated my expertise with a bit of awe. He was the heart patient and I was his doctor. The marsh was different. Here Ezra and I were in each other's hands. The field was more nearly level. I was the greenhorn who needed his expertise to get in and out of the marsh in one piece. I enjoyed his friendship, but I also valued entering an inaccessible wilderness with a master guide. He liked the companionship, but also the reassurance that his doctor was with him and could pull him out of the marsh if need be. I felt a twinkling insight into the patient's predicament—trusting a doctor to get through a dangerous stretch. What was the basis for that trust?

A year earlier, Ezra was hauled out of the marsh in congestive heart failure; a hunting buddy dragged him (reluctantly) to my office on the advice of my senior partner, also on the hunt. Ezra was small and wiry. Used to hard work, he figured his breathlessness was nothing more than "flu." I examined him and told him what I thought was wrong. He registered surprise, but not doubt. Later, as I got to know him, this relatively early trust puzzled me, because I learned just how deeply he distrusted authority. A lot of this stemmed from his real-life experience with overconfident doctors, lawyers, and judges he guided in the marsh. Yet for some reason, he chose to trust me early in our relationship. What accounted for this? Perhaps it was transference of trust from my senior partner, Joe, to me. Was it self-confidence, confidence that he could tell if something I told him didn't sound right? I don't think it was necessarily my wordy explanations of his problem. He told me, "Don't worry about explaining everything. You jus' get me outta this and I'll stick to you like glue." Maybe it wasn't completely rational—something more akin to personal chemistry.

I scanned ahead of the boat for frog eyes and alligator eyes. To my right and left, I saw wide-space amber reflections like little periscopes just visible above the water's surface.

"Doc, we're getting hung up in this algae. You're gonna need to get out and pull us through this."

Surprisingly, my first reaction wasn't to question the logic of getting out of the boat and wading through an alligator-infested marsh. Perhaps my predicament was a bit like the resignation a patient with no good alternative feels when a surgeon diagrams his or her outlandish plan on their abdomen. What were the options? I knew the bottom was too soft to push off with our gig-poles, and I couldn't think of a better idea. I was resigned to our predicament. Moreover, Ezra was just eminently trustworthy to me. Of course I had plenty of reason to trust him—we were close friends by now, and during our many excursions into the marsh he had never steered us wrong. Still, I couldn't help wondering: Was he an alligator expert? He knew this would be safe? I put down my gig, removed the headlight and battery, and readjusted the shoulder straps to my waders.

"What'll the alligators do when I wade ahead?"

"They'll move away. Don't worry about 'em. Keep both hands on that rope tied to the front of the boat. If you step in a hole, your waders'll be fulla water an' sink you like lead. You'll need the rope to pull yourself up."

"You mean an alligator hole?"

"Yeah."

These were 20 feet in diameter and might be 7 or more feet deep this time of year, wallowed out during the dry season. I was glad he pointed this out. It would have been easy enough to drown with waders full of water, and Ezra, with his weak heart, probably wouldn't have been able to pull me out.

I lowered myself over the boat's edge, boots sinking into the mud and waders immediately filling with water. I pulled myself through the mud and around to the front of the boat. Grabbing the nylon rope, I started slowly tugging us forward out of the grass and algae and into open water. Being out in front of the boat felt eerily like going under the knife. I felt a strong urge to focus on trusting Ezra. Without my lamp, I couldn't see light reflecting from the alligators' eyes, but at the surface level I could see the small black silhouettes of their foreheads disappear. Little eddies appeared where their eyes had been.

Without warning, my head slipped under the water; I can only liken the sensation to the moment before anesthesia works, when you give in to trusting that you'll come out on the other side of the experience alive. After a split second of disorientation, I realized that I had stepped over the edge of a hole. My waders, already filled with water, pulled me down a slimy embankment. In total blackness, I focused on not letting the rope slip out of my hands. A thought flashed through my mind: He says the alligators are gone; I'm sure he's right; my legs are intact. I reached the bottom of the hole and began to pull the rope hand over hand until the rope was vertical and the boat directly overhead. I pulled myself part way out of the water and grabbed the bow. I wiped my eyes. Ezra was leaning over the edge, his headlamp on, looking at me; the surgeon was going to tell me that I was still in one piece.

"Hey, Doc, you awright?"

"Yeah. I think we're clear of the grass now. You can use the motor."

I was glad that was over. I climbed into the boat.

Making the Rounds

GEORGE YOUNG, MD

You know her …
skinny, blond, pinched mouth, pinched brow, handshake
like a dead trout, pain
everywhere, making the rounds, to neurologist,
cardiologist, gastroenterologist, psychiatrist, rheumatologist, referred

by her PCP (God bless him)
to you.

She is separated, getting a divorce, can't sleep. System Review lights up
like a pinball machine. Into the ER last week twice
for Demerol for headaches, chest pain.
Scheduled for

an MRI and a treadmill ECG next week. She asks
about Mayo's. You wonder …

would it help
if you could just wrap your arms around her, smooth
the damp tendrils of hair from her temple, kiss
her pale forehead?

No! That is not allowed!

You talk, try to explain, lie a bit, write out prescriptions (being careful
to avoid narcotics) for totally inadequate
medications,
which you know will all cause horrible and bizarre
side effects.

Later, dictating into the system, you ponder
the diagnosis ...

the ICD for unhappiness.

Surveying the Dying: Medical Epidemiology and the Terminally Ill

ERIC AMSTER, BA

We can give them no other information except that we do not know: We do not know where it comes from, we do not know how you get it or why it kills you, but we know that it will. Epidemiologists have determined that here in Mexico most persons with idiopathic pulmonary fibrosis will die within two to three years of their diagnosis. As physicians, we are left to do the only thing we can, which is to ask: "How many months of your life have you lived within the municipal limits of Mexico City? Have you ever seen cockroaches, mice, or rats in your house? Do you have any pets, and if so, what kind and how many? Have you ever smoked cigarettes, cigars, marijuana, or crack cocaine?" We ask question after question, shots in the dark, each seemingly haphazard and misplaced. We write protocols and questionnaires and apply for funding and write reports. The study participants, or cases as they will be ultimately considered, are at the end stage of their disease. Coughing and fibrosing, with looks both of hope and exhaustion, they are dying.

"Have you ever used at any point in your life any of the following to cook with for more than ten hours a week: coal, firewood without chimney, firewood with chimney, natural gas, or propane?" They think back and recall a lifetime of kitchens. Sometimes I think I see a smile when one recalls the use of firewood to make the morning's tortillas, back in another life, another house, before getting married and leaving home for the first time.

"On average, how many hours a day would you cook with it?" A story begins with Sundays, when more tortillas were made. *We cooked nearly all day. Usually we would use twigs from the yard, except for during the rainy season when for months dry wood was scarce and something else, usually coal, was used.*

"Did you do the cooking, or were you present during the cooking?" *We were all there, all my sisters, helping our mother with her work. We each had our own job. As I got older there were more responsibilities, and I would spend more time preparing meals. My daughters help me now in the kitchen. Is that dangerous? Could they get what I have?*

"Did you use ventilation while cooking?" *No. Should I have?*

The study instrument follows with, "Have you at any point in your life worked?" A curious look grows on the man's face as if an impossible question was just asked. He takes a moment to consider what life would be like without work. *Of course,* is the reply, and the number "1" is marked on the questionnaire signifying a positive response.

"Please list all the jobs you have had for over 6 months." His illness forced him to stop working at the age of 78. There are nearly 70 years of jobs to recount since *helping my father sell fruits at the local mercado. I remember being a little kid and helping carry the produce and staying at the market until dark. For most of my life, I have provided for my family by working as a salesman.*

"Have you ever been exposed to any of the following while at work: asbestos, silicon, solvents ... ." *No. Nothing like that. Listen, I sold lots of different things. Some years it was flowers, other years I did well selling books, but I never sold chemicals or anything dangerous.*

"Did you ever work outside on a main street with more than 5 lanes of traffic?" *How could I not? I would sell more during the afternoon rush hour than I could the rest of the day. You sell where you must to provide for your family.*

"Have you or anybody else in your natural (not including godfather), immediate (not including aunts, uncles, or cousins) family ever been told by a medical doctor that you have any of the following: sarcoidosis, asbestosis, alveolitis, scleroderma, Sjögren syndrome … ." *How can I know this! I am a farmer, not a doctor. If I was a doctor, would I understand this question? Would I be sick? Would I be dying?*

In the study instrument, a question like this has three possible responses: No, Yes, and Do Not Know. Because perhaps of fear or pride, the final response is rarely used. Usually a knowing "No" is the only box left to be filled out. Statisticians will inevitably report a population that, despite very little formal education, knows its family history of rare, idiopathic respiratory diseases.

It is difficult for any compassionate physician to see patients in distress. When we feel we are contributing to their distress, difficult situations become excruciating. Epidemiologic research is an integral part of discovering why people get idiopathic diseases, but we must realize that the process of collecting data can further fatigue an already exhausted patient. Intrusive and even culturally inappropriate questions can also compromise trust. Not only is it important to consider the effect this might have on the accuracy of data, but when the investigator is also the patient's physician, the potential effect on patient care is not trivial.

How do you encode a life? Is it possible to assign a collection of life experiences a binary number? How can you correctly assess exposures and risks when you leave out the person, his fears and wishes? Can the sometimes static questions asked of sick cases and healthy controls adequately translate into the understanding of disease etiology? And how can we hope to avoid recall bias when administering an hour-long questionnaire to patients who are extremely tired, weak, and scared? At the end of it all, we are left with an "instrument" filled with 0's and 1's, broken by faded and inaccurate memories, filtered by retrospect and regret.

A Memorable Patient

STEPHEN GOLDFINGER, MD

The few of us who had examined two years of his correspondence before Mr. J.'s arrival at Massachusetts General Hospital were even more interested in meeting the man than in validating the exotic diagnosis we had made from his letters.

Herman J., a native of Rumney, New Hampshire, announced himself to us in March 1958 using a lined sheet of paper, green ink, and handwriting from an earlier century. His request triggered a series of remarkable exchanges with Dr. Charles Clay, our hospital's assistant director at the time. Charlie Clay had grown up in rural New Hampshire within a few miles of Mr. J. Their extensive correspondence occupies a thick section of a hospital record that is still in my hands. The following excerpts depict the improbable relationship that built up between the two men.

Gentlemen, began Mr. J.'s first letter, *I would be pleased to have a little information. What would the cost be for a Appendix Operation if it becomes neccessary? I asked them at Laconia Hospital here in N.H. an I find that nobody can afford to play around with them. I don't have their kind of money at all. Maybe a poor man is supposed to die.*

Enclosed find a stamp for reply.

Yours sincerely,

Herman J.

Within a day, Charlie Clay crafted a reply. (He also penned a brief inquiry to a friend in the region who soon informed him that Mr. J. was a loner who tinkered with guns, sold newspapers, took on odd jobs, and paid his bills on time.)

Dear Mr. J.,

Our regular ward rate is $28 for the first day, $26 for the second, $24 for the third, and $21 a day thereafter, with operating rooms, anesthesia, x-ray and other special services added." After telling Mr. J. of several other hospitals in New Hampshire he could try, he closed by writing, *It is customary for one's own doctor to arrange for admission to a hospital, anyway, as doctors know more about hospitals and their ways than other people do.*

Yours truly,

Charles L. Clay, M.D.

It was Mr. J.'s response that gave us our first intimation of both who and what we were dealing with:

Dear Mr. Clay,

Your letter of March 19 read and contents noted .... I want to say that if doctors don't know any more about hospitals and their ways than you appear to know about yours, they don't know $1/4$ part as much as those other people you tell about. You only gave price of ward 4 days, nothing else. For Pete's sake, how long is a man supposed to be cooped up for an appendix operation—all summer? As for x-rays, I don't see wherein that is needed. You know where to find it, don't you? ... I don't have any doctor as I have not needed one much. I always figured they were a darned good thing to keep away from. There isn't one in a dozen that knows B from bull's foot. It can be truthfully said that a lot of them don't know enough to pound sand straight in a rat hole .... I have not got any need of a Doctor telling me what the trouble is, I am more than satisfied. If I am wrong, I will make a wager. I will suck a dozen woodpecker eggs .... Now my symptoms are the following, not that it will mean anything to you. Go to sleep reading without any warning. Have spells I am slightly dizzy .... Skin on my face feels quite warm and turns red, also the hide on my hands turns red. This leaves in a minute or so, and my face will be white and pinched up for a few minutes .... Right side, very low down is quite sore to the touch. At time it will be sore up above .... I have got more relief from standing on my *head than any other one thing. I figure this trick turns the appendix sac bottom side up an lets the poisons drain off into the intestines. Wish I had got onto this trick earlier. This letter may be frank but you show me where in it isn't 100% right. I thank you for the little information I got which sure was not much. I will guess as to price of the Ether Artist an operating Doctor.*

Yours sincerely,

Herman J.

Thereupon, Charlie Clay committed an act unthinkable for a hospital administrator, even at that time. He prepared a four-page, single-spaced typewritten response to this belligerent eccentric with a bizarre problem. From its first sentence, the letter carries a tone of humility:

Please accept my sincere apologies for the likely delay between my receipt of your letter and your receipt of this answer. I felt that your problem merited my personal attention and offer of assistance. As you see, it required a rather lengthy letter, and I have been under such pressure of work during the past three weeks that I could not get to it before.

Dr. Clay then goes into detail about hospital rates, options for financial assistance, the value of good medical care, and respect for self-reliance. The letter reads as a friend's heartfelt plea for Mr. J. to seek sound medical attention. It gently instructs Mr. J. to start looking around for woodpecker eggs.

The response:

Your long letter of April 10th read an contents carefully noted. I have had 2 or 3 Chiropractic adjustments for Appendix since I wrote you last. Those adjustments coupled with standing on my head to get rid of the poison has already cleared up 85% of my trouble. So I shall not have to look around for the woodpecker eggs. I knew it was a case of appendix trouble and told you so ... .

A six-page harangue on doctors and medical care followed.

As the months progressed, letters kept being exchanged. Dr. Clay described being out of action with an illness of his own. Mr. J. reported continued deterioration and a desire to come to Massachusetts General:

I'm not looking for anything fancy or style. If a surgeon is needed, I of course, would want a good one, naturally. After the job is done you can put me out in the barn in the hay mow if it is warm and comfortable an I can get a little attention now and then ... .

At long last, an admission was arranged, but it never occurred. The sick man explained:

Well in your letter of a while ago you said come down any Monday an I took you at your word. I came down on the 22nd Washington's birthday. I found everything at a standstill. They wouldn't as much as look at me ... .

Dr. Clay wrote a note of deep apology.

A subsequent letter from Mr. J. recounts unrelenting symptoms, despite an appendectomy performed by a local surgeon. He describes worsening of an "evil reddish purple color," a swollen face in the morning, leg swelling during the day that subsides at night, loss of appetite, and a melting of his flesh. He reports a visit to a chiropractor who placed him on a diagnostic machine. Its readout was that he had poisons in his liver.

The response from Dr. Clay was immediate:

I don't know anything about repairing gun actions and you don't know anything about the practice of medicine. The result of our infringing on each other's territory could be disastrous ... . Now for heaven's sake, don't start arguing with me about chiropractors and their machines but get yourself down here as fast as you can and let us begin working with you ... .

On 18 July 1960, some 28 months after his first letter, Mr. J. was finally admitted to Massachusetts General. He was initially bedded in the overnight ward so that we could have the thrill of presenting him to our chief resident. As a member of the team, I observed a craggy-faced, subdued gentleman whose skin colors were on constant display. A panorama of red, orange, and purple shades interchanged from moment to moment, occasionally vanishing into unexpected pallor. His face had permanent telangiectasia, a huge liver could be easily felt, and a systolic heart murmur was audible. No diagnostic machine was needed to diagnose florid carcinoid syndrome. But in a peculiar way, realizing how little we could do for Mr. J., I didn't feel as though we were saying much more than what he had already been told—that there were poisons in his liver. The positive results for urinary 5-hydroxyindoleacetic acid we obtained were hardly a surprise, nor was the report we received from a New Hampshire hospital of extensive carcinomatosis found during the appendectomy in March. Mr. J. endured three weeks of observation and useless treatment at Massachusetts General before returning to New Hampshire to die.

This all unfolded during my first month of internship. To this day, Mr. J. is easily the most remarkable patient I have ever encountered, with a personality as colorful as his disease. Having hauled out his chart once more to reread 40 pages of letters, another thought struck me: Charlie Clay was no slouch as a memorable character either.

Simple Gifts

CHRISTINE S. SEIBERT, MD

It was only my second day as a "real doctor." I was nearly one hour be-hind schedule, and it was only 10:30 A.M. I was already exhausted. Outpatient medicine had seemed so easy six months ago, when I was finishing my residency. How confident I had been then. How insulted I had felt when my clinical judgment needed supervisory approval. Now I wished with all my heart that I could have that safety net back.

I had really done it now. New job, new state, new home, new baby. What was I thinking when I left the "mothership" of my residency, my universe of the past three years?

No time for self-pity. I moved on to my next patient. When I looked at the schedule to find the reason for the visit, I saw "meet the doctor." I was hopeful. How long could it take to meet the doctor?

As I walked down the hallway looking for my yellow and blue door flags, I noticed the most ominous of signs. A stack of charts, nearly knee-high, waited outside the room that held my next patient, Irene. Too much history to squeeze into the usual receptacle for charts. My heart sank. With a deep sigh of apprehension, I left the mountain of manila folders in the hallway, opting to go in empty-handed to as-sess the situation. I braced myself, turned the doorknob with my sweaty palm, and entered.

A very rotund woman, dressed in full Green Bay Packers regalia, greeted me with a huge smile and said, "Welcome to Wisconsin!" She momentarily stopped crocheting to give me a handmade dishtowel, similar to the one she was working on. I must have looked dumbfounded because she explained, "It's for you, a welcome gift." I thanked her and then tried to dig into her obviously complicated medical history. Irene had other plans and proceeded to ask me questions about my background, where I grew up, my education and training, and my family. Apparently satisfied with my answers, she began to pack up her belongings. She had decided our interview was over. Wasn't she going to summarize the volumes of charts outside the door?

Irene said, "Doc, I can see you are busy. I feel great, better than ever. You will have plenty of time to get to know me. I just wanted to be one of the first to welcome you." And with that she departed, leaving me holding my new dishtowel.

That evening, I searched the still-unpacked crates in my new office. I found what I was looking for: a box containing a strange collection of mementos. There was the keychain, *faux* leather, handstitched with black plastic thread, made in a craft therapy session by Peter, a schizophrenic patient I had met on my psychiatric clerkship. There were assorted headbands and barrettes designed by Jack, an entrepreneurial patient who had sent me a carton of the hair accessories after one of his congestive heart failure exacerbations, when I was his ponytailed intern. Buried in the box was the card that had accompanied the most touching of the eclectic group of gifts. That card and several pounds of fish caught off the coast of Maine had traveled with a proud veteran for more than five hours in a Veterans Administration van to be delivered to me in Boston. Joe, the grateful fisherman with heart disease, came dressed in his Veterans of Foreign Wars uniform and ceremoniously presented me with his gift and his thanks for "saving his life." I placed Irene's dishtowel in the box.

My treasures are not fancy or expensive, certainly nothing like some of the gifts I have heard about, the cases of rare wine or the ringside seats to sold-out games. Yet the memories of Joe, Peter, and Jack, along with their humble expressions of gratitude, are the reason I brought this box with me halfway across the country to my new life. Sometimes, after a particularly difficult day, I sift through my box to be reminded of, and sustained by, these special encounters in my journey as a physician.

Pretzels and Fruitcake

KATHRYN RENSENBRINK, MD

It is a peculiar privilege of a rural doctor to walk among one's dead. When I was training in San Francisco, I never thought about the cemeteries. I was too busy analyzing test results and considering treatment options to wonder what happened when my patients went home, or when they died.

In the rural Maine town where I now practice, my patients are also my neighbors. I find myself discussing inhalers in the bakery and clarifying diuretics in line at the supermarket. "Yes, Mr. Randolph, the one that makes you pee." My patients see me in dirty sweats at the Y; they hear my half-muttered invectives to the referee during high school basketball games. I've traded the safety and authority of anonymity for membership in a community.

My way home winds along a country road through fields and woods with occasional startling glimpses of the sea. Only three years in practice, and already the road is crowded with stories. Here lives Susan, who remembers riding to a dance in the town's first motorcar; here lives John, who triumphs slowly over a stroke. And here stands the empty house of Dr. Smith. A physician till the end, he requested his own autopsy, adding "Be sure I receive a copy."

At the curve in the road by the beach lies Bridgett's house. I visit occasionally to enjoy tea and fruitcake, her late husband's favorite. We talk of neighbors, her daughters. When our conversation turns to Dan, her eyes reveal an enduring disbelief that she should be left so much alone. He died at home, a second cancer making merry in a body humbled by the first. "Enough of chemotherapy and transfusions," he'd said, and returned to his view of purple mountains. I made a home visit on his last night. "Is it time?" his family asked. "Are we doing as we should? He was in pain; we gave him an extra pill." I reassured and comforted them, feeling puny before the unknowable. He passed quietly at dawn. Later, his daughter sent a letter thanking me for my visit—"for coming like a guardian spirit out of the winter dark." How wonderful to be most appreciated when you feel the least able.

A bit farther along, I pass Sharon's lovely cottage, where I often slow to avoid her nonchalant cat. I met her in the hospital after her husband, Martin, 50, collapsed in cardiac arrest at a local hardware store. When I picked up the hospital service, he was on a breathing machine, with worsening kidney failure; he had not regained consciousness, maybe never would. I spoke with Sharon and her two children. Did they understand what has happening? Did they know what Martin would want? His intelligence and wit, they quickly agreed, were most important. "We would play six-on-one Trivial Pursuit and he would still win." They laughed, a flash of pride and love sweetening their sadness. I sent him to the tertiary care hospital for an EEG. Shortly after the neurologist had shared her grim prognosis, Martin's heart stopped again, and his brave family let him go.

In the city where I trained, my relationship with these men and their families would end there. I would mull over their fate, evaluate my role, and move on to the next assignment. Not so now. Just before I reach my house, I again pass Dan and Martin, the newest inhabitants of a small cemetery whose stories span three centuries. I like to walk among the quiet white stones, pulled up in neat rows like pews in an invisible church. (Whether it is a church for the dead or for the living, I'm not sure.) At the back, Bridgett has placed a stone bench and planted an herb garden over Dan. Martin lies nearby under a graceful maple. The care given these graves shows me that, though dead, these men remain part of our neighborhood.

I mentioned this thought to Bridgett one day over tea. She then asked if I had noticed the pretzels. Pretzels? "To commemorate the anniversary of my husband's death, my daughter and I walked to the cemetery. After making our tribute to Dan, we visited the nearby graves. We saw what looked like pretzels scattered on Martin. I later asked Sharon if she knew what they were, but she claimed to have no idea." Bridgett's eyes laughed. "I didn't believe her, so I asked again. Finally, she conceded that she had put them there. They had been her husband's favorite." The laugh spread from eyes to mouth as Bridgett went on. "Sharon was mortified—until I told her I only found Martin's pretzels because I was there spreading fruitcake for Dan."

Acne

DANIELLE OFRI, MD, PhD

A young Navajo woman files silently into my office, making no eye contact. As she slips into the chair, errant strands of black hair spill across her face. Through the breaches, I catch glimpses of her rich dark skin riddled with the pockmarks of severe acne. Violently swollen pustules and angry red craters contort the architecture of her face. Her shoulders slope into her slight body, as if afraid to claim too much territory on their own. She contemplates the linoleum wordlessly. I am almost afraid to interrupt.

I am not her regular physician. At this clinic, she has no regular physician because of high turnover and a chronic shortage of physicians. I myself am just a "temp," a hired hand deposited only briefly into this small New Mexico town.

I ask my patient what brings her here. She quietly lays out her litany of symptoms: fatigue, headaches, stomach pains, and her worsening skin condition. I leaf through her clinic chart as she speaks, and I can see that over the years, acne has been her major problem. It is repeatedly noted that she cannot afford to see a dermatologist for specialty treatment.

Almost perfunctorily, I ask my usual question about the presence of stress in her life. Almost as perfunctorily, she replies that her husband hanged himself two months ago. He had made an earlier suicide attempt. Then, their 12-year-old son found him dangling and untied the rope. The father was furious and beat the boy. Four weeks later, the father found the rope his son had dutifully hidden and hanged himself again, this time successfully.

My patient remains impassive as she relates this tale to me. "This is where he hit me the first time," she says, raising her sleeve above her elbow. "The beer bottle was already broken when he hit me, so it left a scar."

I lean over to look where she is pointing—the purple scar is jagged and raised. It has pulled the skin around it into an ugly pucker. The harshly engraved lines remind me of the craggy desert landscape that I see in the morning as I drive to work. I can feel a dry heat emanating from where she points.

"It doesn't show on the stomach," she says in her unembellished monotone, "but I still get pains here." She pulls her shirt up, and I see golden skin with faint stretch marks. "When I was pregnant, I tried not to let him kick me there, but it was hard sometimes."

I don't see scars, but my ears pound with screams.

"I had my tubes tied," she says. "But he was mad; he wanted more kids. I thought two was enough, but he wanted more—'a *real* Navajo tribe,' was what he said." She intertwines one finger in an ebony lock of hair. Her voice continues, flatly, plainly. "He got drunk a lot more then. He wanted me to get another operation. To untie them. It's not that I don't like kids—I love my boys—but I wasn't sure if we should have any more. Kids are expensive." She rotates her fingers, and the hair twists with it, glistening under the office lights. I am beginning to perspire in this overly air-conditioned room.

"Almost a year we argued about it," she says. "We had some bad fights. But I finally decided to do it, untie them. I do like kids. I made an appointment at the hospital for the surgery, but he was mad because it wasn't soon enough. Then he killed himself."

I try to respond matter-of-factly, wanting to put her at ease, but I am assaulted by the vision of a man hanging and a young child stumbling into the room. Was the body writhing in agony? Was the face exploding with hypoxic torment? What did it look like from 12-year-old eyes? What could it feel like to unhitch a rope from a dying man's neck?

"What about my acne?" she asks. "Can't anything be done?"

For a moment I can only blink dumbly at her, fixated on the web that extends far beyond this office and the capabilities of the medical profession. I hunger for powers to untangle the knots, but medical school has not made me a healer of all pains. The illusion of omniscience blithely promised by my residency training is easily deflated by the unadorned actualities of life. Her acne is all I can attack, although I see that physicians before me have waged this war without success.

Surveying the medical history chronicled in her chart, penned by so many different hands, I observe that she has already tried most of the basic acne medications. There is one, however, that she has not taken. It is rarely prescribed for women of childbearing age because of its toxic effects on fetuses—each individual capsule brandishes the image of a pregnant woman with an ominous "X" slashed through the swollen belly—but my patient's plans to reverse her tubal ligation were aborted by circumstance.

This medication is not available in our clinic pharmacy, and my patient does not have the means to obtain it on the outside. I have been told that drug companies will occasionally provide medications without charge. The bureaucracy can be arduous, and there is no guarantee of success, but I think we should try. My patient agrees.

I observe in her chart that she has not had a recent Pap smear. I offer her the option of seeing the gynecologist, but she prefers that I perform it, at our next visit. I am honored.

I watch her padding silently down the hall. Weakly, I retreat to my office. The stout medical textbooks and cabinets overflowing with equipment are stifling, mocking. Where did I get the absurd notion that I might be a healer?

When my month at the clinic is up, I will move on. Just one in a stream of physicians, I, too, will abandon this young woman, bequeathing her only a bottle of pills. I scribble a note to call the drug company and then tape it to my bag. I cannot afford to forget.

Mrs. Posner's Smile

DANIEL R. FEIKIN, MD

She arrived like the others: fasciculating eyelids, cyclic moaning, odor of stale urine. You come to regard them in a certain way. You roll them like logs, reaching in to place your stethoscope over bags of papery skin. You offer them too-loud, semi-facetious greetings, as if their ailment were deafness rather than coma. You identify them by their numbers—sodium, white blood cells, oxygen saturation—and they stand out as notable individuals only by the salient aberrancy of their counts.

The night of her admission, she was a sodium lady. I drew my first blood gas on her. How fortunate I was to do my first on a sodium lady; there were no questions such as "Now, how many times have you done this before?" My resident easily immobilized the woman's arm, which her brainstem made a reflexive attempt to withdraw. Only a slight groan bore witness to the quiver of my hand as it searched for the radial artery. With the flash of red in the syringe hub, she blipped into my medical school history book—"first blood gas." And her entry would have remained at that if it weren't for what awaited us the next morning.

When the team entered her room, she was perched in the bed, her hair matted into a hoary cockscomb. A bland expression hung on her face. The chief resident boomed, "How—are—you—today, Mrs.—POSNER?" I don't think any of us expected the metamorphosis that the question elicited. Her half-mast eyelids drew up, revealing a pair of lively blue eyes. She smiled at the chief in a familiar way, as if he were her grandson. Then she pursed her lips and gazed toward the heavens in contemplation. After a moment she sighed, her eyes engaged the chief again, and, in a voice that was surprisingly robust, she began to respond. Her words were well articulated and carefully chosen, her speech exceptionally fluent.

But it made no sense. A rift gaped between the form and content of what she said. Her statements swung from the illogical to the fictitious. She had lived in this building (the hospital) for years, although she couldn't recall its name. She claimed to have been born in the early 19th century, yet she said that she was 29 years old. The team started to giggle nervously. Her leprechaun eyes seemed to laugh along with us. Perhaps she was toying with us, I thought.

Later that afternoon, the nurses propped her up in a vinyl recliner in the hallway. As I passed her, I stopped—as only a medical student is able—to chat. I explained my role on the team. She seemed interested and even asked a couple of appropriate questions. I left to talk to another patient. Five minutes later, I walked by her again and said hello. A few paces down the hallway, a mischievous thought came to me. I backtracked and asked her if she knew who I was. She scrutinized my face, scanned me up and down, and pronounced, "I have never seen you before in my entire life." After another five minutes, I returned and asked again if she knew me. "Sure, we met in 1949 at the Kit Kat Club."

I had seen stroke patients who couldn't speak or understand, but I had never encountered anyone with a deficit quite like Mrs. Posner's. Even after seeing her severely atrophied brain on the CT scan, I still wasn't sure whether her glib untruths were cortical reflexes or deliberate fakes. I noticed that she used several strategies of engagement. One was outright confabulation. A question such as "What floor are you on?" would be met with an elaborate zigzag involving a brass-plated door, two elevator rides, turning right, ascending twelve steps, and then turning left. Sometimes, she could stymie you with abruptness:

"Where are you?"

"Here."

"What type of building is this?"

"This kind."

On other occasions, your question would produce a furrowed brow and a pensive stare, as if you had just laid the weight of some unsolvable metaphysical question on her. For instance, once I asked her about her parents. She proudly stated their identities as "Melvin and Myrna Cantor ... and I was Sheila Cantor." I asked her why she had changed her name to Sheila Posner. A quizzical pucker usurped her smile. For a long minute, she pondered. Then she locked her eyes on mine and with a resigned sigh acknowledged, *"That* ... is a really good question."

During the week of her hospital stay, I visited Mrs. Posner often. Our conversations would slip away from her within minutes, but she really did seem to enjoy them while they were happening. When she was alone, the expression on her face fell into the blank mask we had observed on the first morning. Yet, when she was spoken to, some switch would click on and she would become cheerful, participatory, and always amusing. I think she knew she was funny. Despite the holes in her memory and logic, she retained an instinct for appropriate context and delivery. One day while I was talking to her in the hallway, a squat janitor approached, pushing a vacuum cleaner. After he passed, Mrs. Posner turned to me and in a completely earnest voice said, "I have known that man for years. And he keeps getting shorter and his butt keeps getting fatter." After pausing for a moment she let out a cackle that made me laugh all the harder.

I can no longer recall Mrs. Posner's sodium level when she arrived at the hospital. I still remember, however, that the morning she left for the nursing home she wore a pink sweatsuit and gold-sequined slippers. Seeing her in that getup made me smile. She smiled back. The world she inhabited was fleeting, stitched together extemporaneously from some retained repository of information. Yet, something essentially human had been preserved. So much so that she kept me guessing right up to that last day. As we smiled at each other, I wondered who was smiling at whom. I think now that enough was still there that we were smiling together.

Vision

BONNIE SALOMON, MD

Your eyes adjust.
Just as in a dark room
Shapes clarify to named things,
Familiar things, a chair, a table, a lamp.

The bruises on a child's thigh reveal
No simple accident, but betrayal.
The scars on arms tell of self-abuse
With needle pricks in hope of a high.
The nervous smile of the teenager
Who took Daddy's car before the crash—
Without permission.

Your eyes adjust
To what hides when light dims:
Courage to get to the next chemo.
The child's been promised a puppy
If he gets through therapy.
When's my poke? He asks,
As though asking for an ice cream cone.

The bravery of a wife of sixty years,
Saying goodnight to her man,
Handsome once in uniform, now
Covered by a hospital sheet.

Your eyes adjust.
Though bereft of light, at last
You see.

A Chapel for Christmas

LOUIS D. BOSHES, MD†

It was early on Christmas Eve, 24 December 1943, and I was far away from home on duty at a U.S. Navy medical facility. I had always requested duty on holidays to cover for my medical buddies who were not of my own faith, and they did the same for me. My patients were a large group of 17-, 18-, and 19-year-old Marines fresh off Guadalcanal, where they had aged rapidly from combat with enemies and tropical illnesses. They were truly ill, both physically and emotionally.

I worked and slept in a little area between both wards heavy with these casualties. That morning, I heard a gentle knock at my door. I called "Come in" and the door opened, revealing two young-old shivering Marines in U.S. Navy pajamas. Both were at stiff attention. Their Atabrine color and their obvious weakness vaulted me from my desk, and I moved them into my quarters and sat them on my bed. I knew them from my rounds as victims of cerebral malaria and battle fatigue. I covered them quickly with my blankets and waited for them to speak, but they remained silent. "Mac. Mac." (We always called the Marines "Mac," except the officers, or we used their first names when we learned them later.) "What can I do for you?"

Dr. Boshes died November 8, 2003.

"Commander, the scuttlebutt has it that you have a shortwave radio. We ain't never been away from home on Christmas—me and my buddy. We were told there was going to be a midnight Mass broadcasted from the States. Could we hear it, sir?"

Immediately I blurted out, "Of course! And I'll come and get you when it comes on. I hope I can bring it in."

"Thank you, sir." They rose to their feet and saluted smartly, but I sent for my corpsmen to wheel them back to their beds.

I knew I had to keep my promise, so I quickly did some thinking. I made some appropriate calls for time factors, learned the proper channels, and then prepared to make my quarters and examining room into a church. I unscrewed a shelf from a wall, covered it with a blanket and white sheet, set it over two buckets, and placed my two pillows on it for kneeling. On a wall, I fastened a small khaki blanket with thumbtacks and in the center pinned a large 18-inch cross, which I had fashioned out of tongue depressors and white bandages. Below this, I placed the radio on a shelf and set lighted air raid candles on both sides. I also placed lighted candles in other areas of my room. From the ward, I brought two Bibles, and laid them at each end of the kneeling board.

Some 15 minutes before midnight, I personally wheeled each Marine to my darkened quarters, lit now only by candlelight. Both gazed silently, yet with amazement, at the holy place I had created out of a bleak military room. Their eyes spoke for them, "Thank you," and my eyes were wet as well. I said, "Here's the radio station you wanted. You've got ten minutes before the start of Mass." I left, leaving the door a little ajar so I could look in from time to time.

For the next hour, the two Marines prayed softly; I even heard sobbing. I made no effort later to talk with them as they padded past me in the darkness back to their beds. Somehow, they had received divine strength.

On Christmas morning, as I made my rounds in the wards, our glances met. No words passed between us, but their glances spelled a lifetime of appreciation. Each squeezed my hand as I passed their beds. I shall always remember those grasps.

I will never forget Christmas Eve 1943, nor will, I believe, those two Marines ever forget that special chapel. That holiday was the emotional high point of my World War II service, a memory I shall always carry with me.

A Time To Listen

DONALD A. BARR, MD, PhD

When teaching my students about what goes into a good doctor–patient interaction, I tell them about the studies that show how quickly doctors interrupt their patients. Male physicians especially, I tell them, are notorious for stopping the patient mid-sentence to redirect the discussion. In one study that I came across, female primary care physicians waited an average of 3 minutes before interrupting the patient to redirect the discussion toward issues more relevant to diagnosis. Male physicians waited an average of 47 seconds.

How long do I wait, I wondered? I decided to try an experiment. I would let my next patient talk as long as he or she needed to explain the reason for seeing me. I would watch the clock and see how long a patient might naturally take to explain the presenting complaint. I would hold my tongue.

The patient was in her 70s and greeted me with a smile as I stepped behind the curtain to be with her. "Hello, I'm Dr. Barr. What's the problem that brings you in today?"

She began to describe the past several weeks of her life. As I recall, it had to do with a coworker noticing something, talking with her sister on the phone, and her reluctance to see doctors. The word "cough" surfaced for a second, then quickly submerged again. Looking at the medicines on the shelf at the drug store and not knowing which to choose. ... Needing to dress warmly ... (Wasn't this weather we'd been having nasty?) ... Sometimes she had trouble sleeping ...

The nurse poked her head through the curtain and silently tapped her watch. The waiting room of our urgent care center was full, and things were starting to back up. I wouldn't budge, though—I turned back to the patient and nodded. However long it took, I would wait for the patient to stop of her own accord. I wouldn't butt in.

It was the cough that was keeping her awake...She always got colds more easily than other people...Her sister was just a worrier ... She finally had agreed to come in to see a doctor, just to reassure her friends and family.

Twenty-two minutes, from start to finish. The nurses were never going to forgive me.

The lungs had left-sided rales. The fever was mild, but the white count suggested infection. The chest radiograph showed a large infiltrate on the left and what I feared was a mass. I called the pulmonary specialist across the street and asked if he could squeeze the patient in that afternoon. He did, only to confirm the worst. It appeared the patient had a tumor causing the infiltrate, and there probably were enlarged hilar nodes as well. She probably had lung cancer, probably in an advanced stage. She needed antibiotics right away to get the infection under control, after which further testing would be arranged.

The patient came back to our center for the antibiotics. The specialist had told her what he had found and had given her an indication of the grave prognosis she faced. I stepped back into the patient's space and said with sadness, "This hasn't been a very good day for you, has it?"

She looked at me for a moment with an unmistakable smile on her face. She reached out her hand and patted me on the wrist.

"Oh, don't worry about all that. I've had a good life. But I just wanted you to know—this is the best doctor visit I've ever had. You're the only one who ever listened."

Twenty Minutes

JOSEPH CAVANAUGH, MD

His was another name to be bellowed out across the waiting room, one of thirteen that morning. But his name gave me pause. Ours is a large public clinic; the waiting room is commodious and always full, and the sound of normal conversation goes nowhere, dies quickly. I hollered his name, came from behind the wall, and shook his hand. He almost smiled or almost winced with our handshake and then sought refuge for his hand in a pocket that wasn't there.

"You made it on time," I observed.

"Yes, I guess. Barely. I try to walk fast when I come here because I know how you are about time, but this heat makes it hard for a body."

He wore drawstring gym shorts tied just below his ribs, and his socks were pulled up to his knees. His shirt, he showed me pinching it off his chest, was wet. There was an apology somewhere in this gesture or in his tone. I put my hand on his damp back both to reassure him and to move him along to the examining room, the press of time upon us. I told him how I loved to sweat, how it made me feel strong and healthy and alive. He nodded absently, his forehead heavily creased, the corners of his mouth pointing down toward his well-trod shoes, and said nothing. I grew bigger in his reticence and pushed the banter, hoping to find the right combination of words that would turn the tumblers and open a door between us.

He groaned barely but audibly as he sat, begging the question that I obliged: "How's the knees?" His knees bothered him incessantly. He walked miles every day, had for the previous 23 months since his wife of 52 years, Rebecca, died in her sleep in the bed next to his. I knew from experience that he wouldn't talk about her because he couldn't find a context large enough. So she remained knotted inside him, rendering him mute.

"Maybe you shouldn't walk quite so much."

"Well, I'm not going to just sit around and think about all of this shit." I didn't know what he meant by "shit," and I didn't ask. In that context, in that room, the word regained some of its lost currency and, coming from him, it was a little jarring. I knew that he had been having sex with a woman 18 years younger than he who lived three floors beneath him and who, by his own account, he hardly even knew, and that this had stirred up a terrible welter of desire and guilt in him. I wondered if this was what he was talking about. Or if he was talking about how every day it seemed a bomb dropped and a village exploded. But I didn't ask because there was so much more to do in the time that we had left. He didn't offer explanations; we had only 15 minutes remaining and he didn't want to be a bother. I was making decisions, prizing forms and required reminders over him, and I knew as I was making them that they were the wrong ones.

His grief was what we would call protracted, pathological. I returned to the knee because time was against us and because, unlike his grief, his knee was a hinge that I could understand. I knew the point about which it turned and approximately how much weight it could hold. The uncaring morning was shouldering past us, and he was sitting there with his undeclared sadness, his throat tied tight against an unending spill of grief. I was both afraid of that kind of grief and painfully aware of the three patients who were waiting and the six more to come later. So we talked about his knees and about his back and a little about the poor fit of his dentures, and he finished a litany of specific, well-rehearsed, utterly familiar complaints. He said, as he always did, "I'm just feeling old, you know, everything hurts when you get old. Don't ever get old." It was his joke, the one he brought out every time. Every time he did he shook his head slowly and his smile arched into a grimace. Every time I thought he was going to cry. What I heard him say was, "Don't think you're ever going to get off easy. Nothing lasts, life is suffering, and there are some things you do when you don't know any better that you will never forgive yourself once you do. Sooner or later your skin will hang off your bones, and your joints will ache from the millions of times you went out to meet your destiny only to have it recede at your approach. You will be alone, if you're lucky enough to be here at all, and you will spend your days avoiding the questions that follow you around because they are your shadow."

He didn't say this, any of this. He just frowned and stared into an empty corner and paused while my eyes took refuge on the computer screen. I glanced at my watch to move things along because when the thing to be said is rude, I communicate nonverbally.

The exam was a ritual, more for me than for him, but he didn't know that. I needed to get my hands on him in order to see him more clearly. I took his hands because I always start with the hands. He offered them to me as fists—the only patient of mine to do this. And although I had no reason to be, I was proud of him for it. I opened his fingers until they were splayed in mine. His skin rolled ridiculously under my thumbs. I cradled his head in my hands, and I asked him to look up as I tugged down on his lower eyelids with my thumbs. Our eyes caught each other for a moment, his clowns' masks of sadness and mine searching and hiding. I draped my left arm across his back and shoulders as a show of solidarity, and almost embracing him from the side, I put my stethoscope on his chest with my right hand and listened to his heart. It stumbled, paused, and then recovered cadence, bandaged and wobbly but still going out to meet the world. Because that is what human hearts do. In that moment, the relentless rush of the morning halted and he and I stood silent, his heart whispering everything he would not say. I opened my eyes as I listened and stared into the perfect furl of his ear.

I returned to my desk and typed a few things into the computer. He returned to the chair beside it and turned his attention again to the corner. I finished typing and was about to recommend a change in his medicine, but when I faced him, my mind changed.

"You must miss her a lot," I hazarded.

He looked at me full on for the first time with a look I did not know. I thought, for a second, that he was going to slap me.

"A lot," he said.

"I know," I said. I didn't. I couldn't possibly.

My job was to advise him about what to eat, about whether to exercise more (or less), and about a prescription for a physical problem. I have been trained for that; for that, I was the authority in the room. At 35 years old, I could offer very little for his real problem. He needed someone to listen to him so that he could tell his story again and again and begin to make sense of it, begin to conclude the story of his marriage and find once more a reason for putting up with all of this "shit." But that would take all day, many days, and our time together was up. He didn't want to see anyone else, someone who might have time for all that needed to be said because, as he put it, "What's the point?" I tried to close with a thought about how some things just take time. My platitudes tasted tinny and stale—even to me as I was saying them—but they were what I had and what I offered. He was gracious about this and accepted them. When we caught each other's eyes for the last time, we both knew that I was saying something mostly because I thought that something should be said.

I love him, I thought, in the conceptual way that I love the guy who peddles fruit on the corner or missing children on a milk carton. More than that. But I resented him a little, too, and for things that were not his fault. We had taken longer than our allotted 20 minutes and "accomplished" little more than completing the required reminders on his record. I felt inclined to tell him this and about the tumult of my emotions for both him and for the system that limits our time and keeps us apart. Like him, I was not sure what the point would be. I didn't know how to effect that relationship without entering into it fully, and I was not sure I had the energy. I knew I didn't have the time. So we parted with all of the unsaid things passing between us in a glance and all of the frustration with our own limitations tugging at us, causing us to linger just a moment longer.

A Medical Lesson

CAROLYN THERESA CLEARY, MD

Half of her smile is sliding off her face—
She blinks furiously to comprehend
What he is saying
As he approaches.
"Good day."
I am the doctor.
I am here now.
"Squeeze my hand—no, stronger."
She blinks more—
Why are you doing this?
But her mouth can't
Form the words.
He smiles pleasantly,
Isn't it grand to be part of this humanity?
"Note, students,
the Babinski reflex."
Half of her begins to struggle
To sit up and see
Who exposes her,

And why.
Meanwhile her neighbor,
Compatriot in age,
Stares blankly forward,
As the phone rings and rings.
The words are there
Her lips can form them—
Doctor save me!
Have you come to deliver me?
But the gurgle which results
Is not noticed by the doctor
As he walks away smiling,
Speaking of
Vessels, and strokes,
And hearts that won't pump
In the night.

The Sharer

KARL LORENZ, MD

The shadowy, dark head, like mine, seemed to nod imperceptibly above the ghostly gray of my sleeping suit. It was, in the night, as though I had been faced by my own reflection in the depths of a somber and immense mirror.

Joseph Conrad, *The Secret Sharer*.

A wall of medals, like multicolored chain mail, clothed Master Gunnery Sergeant's bulging pectorals. He was polish and shine from his balding pate to his oil-slick black uniform shoes. The creases in his pants and shirt were as sharp as a knife's edge and as freshly pressed as a groom's going-away suit. His few short hairs stood at perpetual attention. He was calm and polite.

I was a lieutenant, and my military experience was limited to a military residency. Master Gunnery Sergeant possessed the most senior enlisted position on our large Marine Corps base. His medals commemorated duty on every continent. "Yes, Lieutenant," he would answer. He was respectful, but I felt ludicrous. He was Experience; I was Ingenue.

Master Gunnery Sergeant was diabetic. I interviewed him and reviewed his records. His diabetes was uncontrolled, and results of urinalysis suggested early kidney disease. He had hypertension, and he was a smoker. After I examined him, we had a frank discussion. We formed a tentative partnership.

Master Gunnery Sergeant's next visit followed my promotion. "Congratulations, Commander!"

"Thank you, Master Gunnery Sergeant. It took long enough!"

My promotion had been delayed for a geologic epoch of military time. I was thankful for Master Gunnery Sergeant's enthusiastic acknowledgment, although my lieutenant commander bars were dubious authority next to his rainbow of ribbons.

Master Gunnery Sergeant started visiting me more frequently. He was preparing for complex oral surgery and dental implants. He announced the plans for surgery with a smile; several gaps were visible in the floor of his mouth where new bone would be grafted. "I guess I'll have to give up smoking," he grinned.

Although his oral surgery was difficult, it forced him to restrict his diet and he quit smoking. Some of his dental implants did not survive the first graft attempt, and his subsistence on pabulum was prolonged. During the next few months, he lost weight and his diabetes improved. We celebrated our fortuitous victories over diabetes and addiction.

On a subsequent visit, he seemed embarrassed and broached the subject of impotence with me. "It's ahhh, difficult, sir. It's not what it used to be, and the wife and I were wondering what you could do." We concluded that the impotence was caused by diabetes, and we discussed a prosthesis and other solutions. I was glad that Master Gunnery Sergeant could trust me with what was obviously an embarrassing problem. I felt a growing camaraderie with my patient.

Master Gunnery Sergeant maintained his abstinence from smoking, but when his oral surgery was complete, I noticed an increase in his fasting glucose level and weight. "Sir, it's a weakness for cake and ice cream," he confessed with a perfect smile. I smiled, too, as I admitted my hidden passion. I indulged the memory of the recent pleasure of a mellow, aged pinot, homemade polenta layered with Bolognese meat sauce and béchamel sauce, and chocolate mousse. What was a piece of cake and some ice cream between friends?

I had been Master Gunnery Sergeant's physician for a year when I asked him about his experience in Vietnam. I had been reading *Dispatches*, by Michael Herr, and I wondered if Mastery Gunnery Sergeant could confirm its dehumanizing account. "Yes, sir. He captures the experience well."

I was amazed; the book's brutal accounts of battle and the cheapness of human life seemed cartoonish. "If you like that, I'll bring you a better book, *Never without Heroes*. It describes the recon experience in Vietnam, and I was recon. At night after reading it, I'd wake up in a cold sweat dreaming that I was fighting Vietcong. It's the best book I've ever read about Vietnam."

I eagerly awaited Master Gunnery Sergeant's next visit. He dropped off *Never without Heroes* and asked me if I had a few minutes. "I don't have many pictures of my time in Vietnam, but I brought you what I've got." Master Gunnery Sergeant pulled a handful of photographs from his pocket like a tourist at homecoming. I expected photographs of liberty hours in the Philippines or Okinawa.

War paint and combat gear adorned a group of smiling teenagers, including a youthful Master Gunnery Sergeant. A dirt trail stretched into the jungle, and pimply faces grinned at the camera. A pit in the center of the trail was filled with charcoal. One of the kids was holding up a lump. The lump had sockets for eyes, and rotting, charred flesh clung to its cheeks. Several other bodies were tossed haphazardly into the pit like back-alley refuse. "That's the Ho Chi Minh Trail, Commander. We'd find those bodies out there, and we'd inspect them to bring back evidence of enemy activity.

"You know, the strangest things would happen out there, Commander. Sometimes when we got into a firefight with a group of Vietcong on the Trail, you'd look down after it was over and realize you'd had an orgasm. That happened to all of us. It was something to do with the intensity of battle." I looked quizzically at Master Gunnery Sergeant.

Photograph number two showed a group of celebrants, their mirthful expressions undiminished by the image's age. The kids looked laughingly at the camera, and two of them held up a trophy, like hunters holding up a buck on opening day. Their trophy was a human corpse, missing its entrails and the interior of its chest. One of the kids held the Vietnamese head by the hair so that its eyes and lips were pulled back and it seemed to smile. Another kid had his free hand stuck through a hole in the dead man's back and was giving the finger to the camera through a bloodied chest wall.

The few remaining photographs were limited to relatively innocent pictures of young men in fatigues and camouflage paint. I reviewed them and thanked Master Gunnery Sergeant. I sat quietly after he left and stared at the comforting wilderness of the surrounding base.

Master Gunnery Sergeant's experience with death in Vietnam was more immediate and threatening than anything I had ever witnessed. I reflected on the contrast between his calm outward demeanor and the violence documented in the photographs he had casually shared with me. I had increasingly come to identify with his concerns and foibles. To the extent that I could empathize with him, I felt that we were alike. Was my empathy misplaced?

I read *Never without Heroes* a few weeks later on vacation. In Lawrence Vetter's vivid firsthand account of battles and reconnaissance patrols, I experienced the barbaric random violence that commingles the blood of ordinary men in combat. In Vetter's detailed stories of inexperienced young men swept up in sudden and unexpected battle, I came to understand the personal terror that is part of war. I read about ordinary men who were capable of extraordinary violence.

Master Gunnery Sergeant invited me to his retirement ceremony in the spring. I missed the ceremony, and I left the Navy shortly after his retirement. Although I no longer have the pleasure of his visits, I think of him often.

A memory: I enter a plain white clapboard church sheltered under towering North Carolina hardwoods. Seated in an oak pew, I gaze at the trim young preacher behind the simple wooden podium at the front. "Anyone who is angry with his brother will be subject to judgment." I shift uncomfortably in my seat. "It is better for you to lose one part of your body than for your whole body to be thrown into hell." I earnestly try to avert my eyes from the coeds, whose dresses dance teasingly in the fall breeze on the church doorstep. I make my way back to the dorm to study and hope that the words of Jesus are metaphorical.

In the main hallway of the VA Hospital where I now work, veterans whiz about like actors in a macabre divine comedy, a motley collection of metallic wheelchairs and human beings with maimed and missing limbs. Is this scene a legacy of random violence, or is it a divine symbol? It reminds me that my own penance is incomplete. I recall the faces in Mastery Gunnery Sergeant's photographs. Every day I am more certain that they would have included my own.

The Man with No Heart

ARI MOSENKIS, MD

As I was en route to the parking lot on a cold autumn night, my pager started beeping. I was a new renal fellow on call, and this was an all-too-familiar, yet still unnerving, occurrence. The number to call back was one I didn't recognize: the OR. When I returned the call, I learned that a heart transplant had failed with disastrous complications. The patient was hypotensive and grossly volume overloaded. The transplant team was requesting intraoperative dialysis.

Minutes later, after probing unfamiliar corridors, I arrived at the scene. By perusing the patient's chart, I learned more about him. He was 47 years old and had a dilated cardiomyopathy. He had been in the hospital for more than 2 months, was dependent on intravenous inotropes, and was awaiting a heart donor. Early that morning a match had been found. The donor was a 20-year-old man who had died of head trauma sustained in a motor vehicle accident.

To enter the OR I had to "scrub in," something that I had not done since my surgery rotation as a medical student. The environment in the OR was tense. I obtained more of the patient's history: The operation had been proceeding well. However, after the new heart was anastomosed in place and the aortic cross-clamp was removed, the situation changed drastically. The donor's right and then left ventricle failed. An intraoperative biopsy showed hyperacute rejection of the donor heart. The patient developed hypotension that was unresponsive to pressor agents. Despite the use of a right ventricular assist device, an intraortic balloon pump, and a left ventricular assist device, the patient remained hypotensive. He was then restarted on cardiopulmonary bypass via an extracorporeal membrane oxygenation (ECMO) device. Yet he was now severely acidemic and volume overloaded. I instructed the perfusionist to insert a dialysis filter in his ECMO device to create a continuous arteriovenous dialysis circuit. The patient was brought back to the cardiothoracic surgical intensive care unit in extremely critical condition. His chances for survival were slim.

I visited the patient the next morning. From a distance his room epitomized "intensive care": wall-to-wall artificial organs. How many organ systems had failed? His old heart was in a bucket in the surgical pathology department, his new heart was a flaccid sack, his lungs were filled with fluid, and his kidneys had completely shut down. Yet when I approached his bed, he looked at me, smiled, and waved. Despite all that his body had endured the previous night, he had sustained no obvious neurologic injury. Subsequently, a neurologist also did not detect any motor, sensory, or cognitive deficits.

Debate still lingers in many circles about the definition of death: brainstem death or cardiovascular death. According to the proponents of the former definition, a person is considered dead when the brainstem dies, even though the most vital of the brainstem functions, breathing, is easily and effectively replicated by a machine. Such was the case with the young man who had donated the heart that my patient's body had rejected. According to proponents of the latter definition, death occurs with the cessation of heart and circulatory functions. How, then, would the proponents of this definition classify my patient? His circulation and oxygenation were being artificially preserved with the ECMO device. Arguably, my patient's situation was no different from that of any patient in an OR undergoing cardiopulmonary bypass. However, his situation was different for two reasons. First, ECMO replaces heart and lung function for several days or longer, as opposed to the more transient nature of intraoperative cardiopulmonary bypass. Second, he was awake and cognitively intact. Certainly, by *any* definition, this man with no heart was alive.

The patient was put at the top of the list of heart transplant recipients. Could anyone have been more critically ill than he? Fortunately, a new donor was found two days later: a 33-year-old man who had died of a self-inflicted gunshot to the head. The second transplant was successful, and my patient slowly improved. Ten days after his first transplant, he was extubated and switched from continuous to intermittent dialysis. An aggressive regimen of physical therapy was initiated. Nine days later he was no longer dependent on dialysis. One month after his first transplant and after more than three months in the hospital, he was discharged home without tubes or wires, without artificial kidney, lung, or heart.

Figuratively, we view the heart as the seat of courage. From this perspective, one thing is evident. My patient, who had endured so much with immense strength, perseverance, and courage, *did* have a heart all along: worn, dilated, and full of life.

On Aging

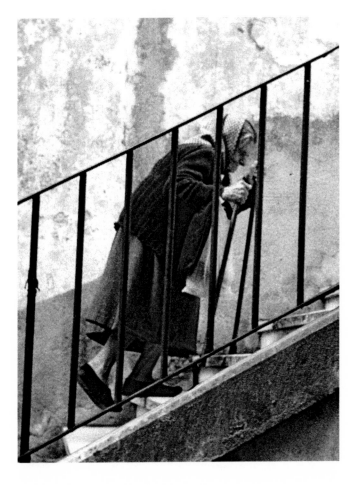

The Aftermath of a Fall

KEIKI HINAMI, MD

As I helped him keep his balance, my grandfather lifted his leg unsteadily. The stench of urine in the train station stall was overpowering. My grandfather, aged 88 and incontinent, had wet himself on the train. I fortunately had packed an extra pair of pants, which I was now struggling to get him into. Even as an older man, he had not been helpless. He had been robust, solo-hiking the tallest peaks of Japan at age 65, teaching me to play ice hockey at 77, and even holding out until 85 before retiring from his profession as carpenter. The transformation into this declining, embarrassed old man was astonishing.

Kneeling on the tiles of the foul public restroom, I did not seek his eyes. I was fighting hard to find a way to guard his dignity. I kept my eyes low, watching him only to make sure that he did not tip over. But our eyes had to meet eventually when I finished tightening the belt around his pants, too large on his lean waist. When I peered up, his eyes were still downcast. He dropped his shoulders, then furrowed and lifted his brow, giving an expression that was unmistakably apologetic. As in a kid who senses guilt after spilling his juice, the contrition in my grandfather's expression evoked sympathy. Or maybe pity. I sought for something to say, something to let him know that everything was all right. I rolled up the soiled pants, took his arm, and together we left the station stall.

These moments I spent with my grandfather were awkward to say the least. I felt remarkably clumsy because there was nothing I could do to make him not feel ashamed. The humiliation of a grown man wetting his pants was too obvious to mask with kind words or thoughtful gestures. I could only resign myself to acknowledge two things in that moment. The first was that the eventual decline of our physical and emotional integrity is inevitable. It happened even to this very strong man. Second, compassionately attending to him may have been the most that I could have done. Stripping him naked neither preserved nor protected his dignity, but it affirmed his significance to me even when circumstance wrested his dignity from him. When there was no poise left in him even to pretend, simply attending to my grandfather distinguished him from any other old man. Moreover, aiding the person within his ailing body allowed me to see his heroic struggle for dignity in light of unchangeable human frailty.

Since this happened a year ago, I have been receiving news of grandfather's deteriorating condition. I see in my daily encounters with the elderly in the hospital how abruptly their lives can change. Falls often cripple and sometimes even herald death for the infirm. Death becomes unavoidable as bodily functions are lost one by one.

Healers must believe in the nobility of the human struggle against debility and dying, but fear and shame are emotions naturally occurring towards the end of a long life. My grandfather, like many of the very old, endures the indignity of falling apart. I am powerless to prevent him from further decline. I can only prevent him from falling alone.

Tell Me

GEORGE YOUNG, MD

Tell me the night silence
on the locked Alzheimer's ward is broken
by a yell from room 206,

that an old man with flattened
nose and crumpled ears,
whose family moved away to Arizona,

whose doctor never comes
to visit, is standing
in the middle of that room, naked,

his freckled face a clenched fist,
urine and feces running
down his legs.

Then tell me that the fat one, twelve
years on the job,
working her second shift because

someone's *car won't start,*
comes with a pan
of warm water, a sponge and a towel;

how, back in bed, he
cries, *You know—*
I'm in the ring tomorrow with Killer;

how a tiny smile begins, how
her hand reaches out
to flick down his wild flame of hair.

Now tell me again
why you don't believe in angels.

Shower Time

MICHAEL D. MARTIN, MD

He sat at a small table covered with a white vinyl cloth and adorned with a vase holding a purple plastic flower. Across from him in a wheelchair was an ill-shaven man he had never seen before. Around him were more strangers, mostly aged and appearing to be in various stages of poor health. There was a lot of noise in the room.

He was a rather small, trim man with determined eyes and snow-white hair, and he sat erect in his chair. He dabbed at the corners of his mouth with his napkin and then with deliberation folded it neatly across his lap. He wore a faded blue cap with a gold British Open logo on it. The man had been an accomplished amateur golfer in his younger days. He had even considered making a run at the professional tour after finishing college, but with a wife and two children to support, the dream was put aside and he became a math teacher. Golf had not been in his thoughts for years but he liked the cap.

A large black woman who looked vaguely familiar was clearing his dishes, and she smiled at him. "You ate good tonight, Mr. Martin. I don't know how you stay so skinny eating as much as you do." He smiled back but didn't answer. His mind was years and miles away. Try as he might, he just couldn't figure things out. Everything seemed backward or upside down or something. In a way this felt like home but this wasn't home, damn it. He wasn't old like these other people, and he had a wife and kids and a job to go to. He was probably late for work already. He was a man who had always taken his responsibilities seriously. He had lots of things to do, and no one seemed to understand. He felt anxious.

He became aware of a hand on his left shoulder, and there was a young lady dressed all in green saying, "Time for your shower, Mr. Martin." He was already late for work, and he didn't have time for this. He didn't *need* a shower, and he sure as hell didn't need help from this girl. He resisted her efforts to ease him out of his chair. He had always had a bit of a stubborn streak and it was showing through now.

A big man appeared, and he felt an uncomfortable tightening around his right arm. Panic took hold of him, and with surprising strength and agility for his age, he wrested from their grasp, bounded from his chair, and backed away from them, fire in his eyes and chaos in his brain.

The girl approached him slowly with soothing tones. "It's just a shower, Mr. Martin. It won't hurt, and it'll help you to relax." Her words were gibberish to him, and he seized her outstretched arm and twisted it with such force that she cried out. Suddenly powerful arms encircled him like tentacles, and no matter how hard he twisted and kicked, he could not break free. He was dimly conscious of a crowd gathering around him and then of a cool moist feeling on his shoulder, punctuated by a sharp jab.

The medicine burned but he didn't notice, and a chemical quiet slowly blanketed his brain. Darkness forced an uneasy truce between inner and outer realities and gradually his body ceased to struggle. Shower time would have to wait as more strong arms hoisted his feet, and he was carried to his room, minus the blue cap, which lay by the table where the man in the wheelchair was finishing his dessert.

Like Snail

GEORGE N. BRAMAN, MD

And then the whining school-boy, with his satchel
And shining morning face, creeping like snail
Unwillingly to school.

Shakespeare, As You Like It

Intrepid snail, spiraled like a volute,
At my doorstep, imperceptibly paced,
Blended with earth like solvent and solute,
How have you been so magically placed?
Just as my step has slowed, my brain grown cold,
My pen's fluency stalled, do you appear,
With steady, snail-like progress, brave and bold,
Gliding dauntless through autumn of the year.
Spurning the flurry of the harried world,
Resolute in your small unerring course,
Your pace defies armies with flags unfurled
Or potentates with chariot and horse.
Like snail, I'd persevere and soldier on
Till brain and heart and fluency are gone.

Changing Diapers at the VA Hospital

JASON DAVID EUBANKS

I am too young
To be father to such an old man—
Too smooth of face,
Too ill-fit for a short, white coat
He thinks able—
Capable to finger
The fragile pride of a blind man
Who once roared his eighteen wheels
Through the mountains of western Pennsylvania—
Winding roads, his Cherokee partner,
And stories of truck stops and prostitutes
Who undressed this man as I now do
As he tells us how he soils his pants,
A grown man who has lost control,
Eighteen wheels of a lifetime's freight
Racing down, looking for a run-off—
Will this white coat ever fit well enough
To help a man become an infant again?
To wrap a diaper around impotence?

Changing Diapers at the VA Hospital

He and I,
Reduced to the same—
Two lives learning
How to put a diaper on.

On Rounds

JERALD WINAKUR, MD

When will my eyes
be as vacant as his

my pulse as weak
my joints as stiff

when will I need
my first walker

first wheelchair
has the cell

that is parent
to my cancer

already mutated
are there now two

four, eight, sixty-four
have they broken
ten thousand
when will my heart

beat in that peculiar
way, require a jump-start

when will it—once
and for all—stop

when will my skin take
on that waxen look

in certain light
it looks that way now

when will I forget
your name

my own?

She is a Beautiful Lady

SARA SASHA BATTAR, MD

Dean, 87, and his wife Donna, 78, would ritualistically arrive every 3 months in my geriatrics clinic, rain or shine. They had been married for 61 years. They lived in the same home for all these blissful years and took great pride in that. From the beginning, Donna ably presumed the spokesperson's role and impressed me as a reliable and caring informant who knew Dean more than he knew himself. These interactions spanned over 4 years. The staff became accustomed to the couple's regular presence and even grew quite fond and sympathetic of their changing dynamics and physical, functional, sensory, and mental declines.

Eventually, Donna reported Dean's progressive forgetfulness and impaired comprehension and retention of important elements of daily life. One of the defining moments in their long and harmonious marriage seemed to involve an incident at a family reunion. Dean failed to recognize their 8-year-old granddaughter Amy and evidenced absolute lack of knowledge about another newborn grandson. This devastated the first-time proud parents, and Donna, of course, but Dean was immersed in a blissful oblivion.

The following clinic visits witnessed Dean's deepening dementia. Donna's stubbornness as an intensely passionate wife, caregiver, and woman of pride would not allow her beloved husband to be taken care of by strangers outside of their home. She was equally opposed to the idea of both of them moving into an assisted-living facility. She was too attached to their home, the memories, the mementos, and their social connections. She was also intensely attached to their local connections—the church, the grocery store, and their neighbors. No amount of persuasion from her daughters, from the interdisciplinary team members, or from me could convince her to reconsider. In every discussion, Dean would pleasantly and willingly allow Donna to tighten and loosen her clasp on his fingers and lock his gaze with hers. Often it would baffle me as to how he could watch the whole process of these discussions centering on him with such a detached stance. There were moments when I wished I had Dean's incredible capacity for detachment myself. With a nonchalant and determined voice, Donna might wonder aloud if the Mayo Clinic perhaps could help Dean's memory.

With understandable reluctance, Donna eventually agreed for home-based primary care services. The home care staff, not surprisingly, relayed to me Dean's worsening memory and activity levels. He remained pleasant, Donna still possessive of him, both determined that they would remain at home. Dean began to feel quite insecure after spending even a few waking moments in Donna's absence. Donna grew frustrated at not having the mere privacy of her bathroom. At such times, Dean would scream for her like a toddler searching for his parent. From a charming, well-sculpted lady who almost always prompted a second gaze from passersby, Donna had become the personification of an elderly, fatigued, and burdened lady with a single mission in life, taking care of Dean.

But Donna never reported any of this during their clinic visits. She had heard enough of friendly reprimands about caregiver burnout, support groups, and specially designed programs for such patients and their families. Somewhat miraculously, however, she permitted us to offer Dean respite care provision in our nursing home care unit for 2 weeks. Dean, with his memory impairment, had no perceivable problems. When Donna visited him 3 days after his admission, she was distraught at his response to her presence. She seemed quite disappointed that he did not miss her or panic in her absence. Worse still, he seemed only vaguely familiar with her and would not call her by her name. Donna's emotions flooded. There was no stopping her. She complained that he had grown worse with the hospital stay and immediately took him home.

Soon Dean lost the memory of his relationship with Donna, which in turn deflated her passion and purpose in life. Dean began to miss his follow-up appointments. The family reported that Donna had an unexpected fall at home. She was hospitalized, and a few days later, she passed away.

Their daughter told me this: "Dad had no reaction and seemed not to acknowledge Mom's death. We explained it to him several times. My 10-year-old seemed to know much more of what had happened than my Dad. Mom was embalmed and looked so very beautiful. We draped her in a gorgeous olive green satin dress with sequins and rich embroidery. She looked so stunning. We took Dad to her casket. He appeared perplexed. He was vaguely familiar with her face, but could not recognize his life partner of 61 years when she was still and motionless, without her apron, without her hovering. He looked at her and returned to his seat. No expressions still. When we asked him, 'Daddy, what did you see?' Dad simply said,

'She is a beautiful lady.'"

Cub Scout Jubilee at St. Cabrini Nursing Home

HAROLD W. HOROWITZ, MD

Lads dressed in blue and gold
framed by the flashing lights
of the Christmas tree
in front of the baby grand
bleat holiday tunes
some mumbling, others talking,
most not knowing the words hum
not yet able to read,
those with colds hacking, sneezing,
none of the age when voices change
and play havoc on any semblance of tune.
Pianist and scout mother
banging and pleading, lift their voices
to give structure to this rush of sound,
so that some words or perhaps
fragments of a passage can be recognized
"Deck the halls with boughs of holly,
fa, la, la, la, la, la, la, la, la, la
we wish you a Merry Christmas dreidel,

dreidel dreidel, I made you out of clay"
like waves crash one after another
without beginning, middle, or end.
The audience, earthbound in this
profane purgatory, held innocently
for sins they cannot recall, wait
as if they had all the time in the world
immersed in this youthful display
of valor and vigor, "We'll do our best,"
with eyes watering and transfixed smiles
heads bobbing on caved in chests
they hear the voices of angels,
and captivated they tremble
no two beats in time
like living ragtime dolls
hands and heads, knees and feet
they are mad conductors coaxing
this choir to make ethereal music,
and how the lads respond in kind
to this cacophony of movement,
it is their duty, is it not?

Dilapidation

CLAYTON J. BAKER, MD

As dirty off-white as
the gray-brown snow melting
in pocked drifts surrounding,
she looks more decrepit
than she actually is.

Weathered paint peels in patterns
along her warped clapboards
suggesting strong, skeletal
squared rough-hewn crossbeams
under blasted facades.

Her balustrade's finer
than any carved nowadays,
tall windows too, stained glass
inlaid atop, each an iris trained
skyward in its upturned eyeball.

But no doubt is allowed by
signs sunk in her front lawn,
her great barn demolished.
Tract housing is coming,
prognosis is dismal.

Why not enter, excise
her carved fireplace mantle,
majestic front door or that quaint
clawfoot bathtub, an organ donation
from doomed house to our house.

Or resect her stout furnace
and transplant it in our
cachectic, kind neighbor
whose body's consumed by
one rogue cell's mad offspring.

If such magical theft would
give her and her husband
one last spring together,
this nine-tenths dead farmhouse
would grant one more harvest.

Rheumatic

D. A. FEINFELD, MD

The serpent-god has cursed her hands
to slither sidelong forever, never caress,
only to grope past each instant,
old loves beyond her painful reach.
The hands curl round her walker's handles
like vines struggling up a fence;
if tendrils untwist and again run straight
they might reach again for needle and cloth.
She moves the cage forward, plants
its four pads the way a cat lands.
The floor comes to a fork: she fights
indecision, groans ahead,
paths lighted by flickers of pain
that harden her limbs to driftwood.
Long nails gnarled into unwanted fists,
she tries to unclench fingers that bend
like a beam passing through time's glass.

The Iridescence of Old Ladies

JOHN McCLENAHAN, MD

When she was 74 years old, Mrs. V. withdrew to Heavenly Rest in suburban Philadelphia, a flat, tidy nursing home of cinderblock design calling to mind a small hosiery mill. Parking is provided. A bed of marigolds, a glassed-in vestibule, gray linoleum, Naugahyde settees, a receptionist in a cerise smock. The air is close, faintly ammoniacal. Inhabitants align the walls in wheelchairs, some drowsy, some in an attitude of listening. The women's hair is thinning; their cheeks pale as white candles. Men wear gray wrappers, exposing their knees.

I'm issued a pass and directions to Room 147. A nurse's aide meets me in the hall. "Most days she's pretty good," she says as we walk to the far end. "Quiet like, you know, but now and then she flies off the handle quicker'n you can say Jack Robinson. You can't make out what she's talking about. Not many people come to see her. Her lawyer comes sometimes."

Mrs. V.'s furnishings are sparse: a cross on the wall, a maple bureau, a bed draped with a green coverlet, a commode, two get-well cards on the windowsill, a walker, a flickering television.

She was one of my first patients: well-born, feisty, loyal. A flirt. She came to me with her most trifling complaints—perhaps, I secretly hoped, as an excuse to chat. Slender, elfin, twice a year outside my office door she parked her Ford station wagon—one of the old numbers with cedar bulwarks—and without a word laid a box of Godiva chocolates and a fifth of Wild Turkey on the table. Sometimes she loitered: "John, would you take some x-rays of my chest and give me some idea of how long the guarantee has to run?"

She lived in a Georgian mansion close by the track of a boy's school where she jogged half a mile every day in her turquoise sweat suit, a sight to stop traffic. Every year on January 17th, Benjamin Franklin's birthday, she invited me to tea in her drawing room amid threadbare curtains, begrimed ancestral portraits, and a lithograph of the Empress Josephine. We nibbled lace cookies from the Acorn Club and exchanged gossip about scandalous Philadelphians. She was a geyser of genealogy. When asked, "Where did Mr. So-and-So's money come from?" she would light a Chesterfield, sit back, gaze at the ceiling, and frown. A nod of recognition. "Oh, yes. It was his third wife but one...." I filled my journal with her remarks, negligently uttered and cast aside. "The only tragedy is not to be loved." "I adored the cats of Alhambra—so lithe, so tawny." "A love affair should subside with grace like the end of rain or descent of a tango. But there are always the dregs...."

Friends of mine stopped at her home one Halloween for trick-or-treat. It was late. They banged on her door and she appeared in her robe, hair in curlers, her face creamed, wearing a chin strap and mask. She greeted them. "Come in, children; *do* come in. As you see, I'm in costume, too!" Once at a banquet, twitted by friends for the size of her diamond solitaire, she took off her glove and pressed her hand into it, remarking to her ring finger, "Now that's enough, George; back into the garage."

A work in progress—a geisha *manquée.*

Presently, to her keen embarrassment, she got lost on her walks in Wissahickon Park and forgot engagements. "My mind isn't lost," she told me, "I've just misplaced it." Her daughters brought her to Heavenly Rest, where she sits at her window and waits, unburdened by reason or regret. I take her hand and she frowns, drawing it away. I dangle bits of information for her approval: the gowns worn last week at The Assembly, the Mayor's recent speech, the opening of a musical on Broadway, the Silver Cup her nephew won at the Sunnybrook golf tournament. Nothing ruffles her indifference. I kiss her and say good-bye, mourning the elegance locked deep in a dark vault.

On Death and Dying

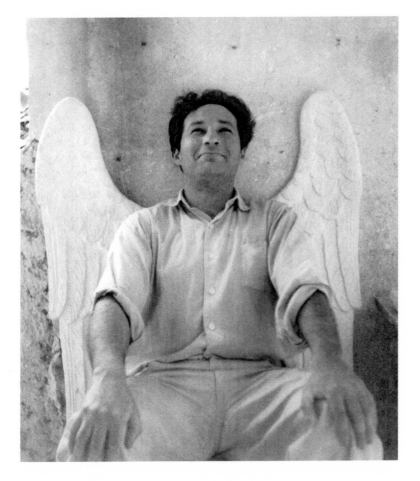

The Woman from County Meath

FRANK BRENNAN, MBBS

The warmth of the Dublin day caught everyone by surprise. Through the window I could see children playing in the garden. The nurse and I walked into the visitors' room. The family was waiting. They were from County Meath. He was a farmer, only 54, she a teacher; they had seven children. It was clear that he was dying. He had battled seemingly intractable pain but now was more settled.

I spoke about the past few days and what to expect from this point onward. I then concentrated on the family themselves and recommended, as we do, the usual things: that family members take turns being with him, that they try to eat and sleep, that they talk to each other, in short that they look after themselves through this vigil. I turned to the patient's wife and said, "I know you've been here all the time over the last few days. It might be good to go and have a rest, even just for a little while."

There was a long silence. She looked at me as though down a passage. She turned her head to one side, looked out the window, then towards me again and said, "No, I will not be leaving him."

She spoke tenderly of their first meeting at age 17, of their courting and wedding day, of their marriage and the birth of children. She spoke in soft beautiful phrases, then sentences that began plainly but became brilliant, each seemingly more evocative than the last. And with every memory of their life together, each reflection she would end by saying, "No, I will not be leaving him," until that phrase, repeated, became the tolling of a distant bell. And then she said something that I had never heard expressed in the same way before. She said that from their wedding day they were united, that they were, as the prayer states, one body, and that as he had fallen ill so had she, that as he was buffeted by the storms of pain so was she, that as he was suffering so was she, and that as he lay dying so was she. No James Joyce, no Oscar Wilde, no Samuel Beckett could have put it so powerfully. As Angela Murphy, the palliative care nurse with me in the room that day, said later, "She was *saying* what he was *feeling.*"

In many ways, of course, she wasn't talking to us. She was speaking across the vast sea of their lives. I had spoken at a practical level about rest. The response I received was from a person adrift on that sea, not wanting to leave or soften the fate.

Too often, as doctors, we speak practically and are heard emotionally. And, perhaps, that is our role.

Angela and I left the room and walked back to the ward. We were both too moved to say much. Later that day, Angela rang me and said, "Frank, we may never hear the like of that again." When I returned to Australia, I was asked to present some memories from Ireland. I contacted Angela. Without prompting she said, "Of course, you'll talk about the woman from Meath." And in distant years, if I were to ever encounter Angela Murphy again, walking down O'Connell Street in Dublin or perhaps George Street in Sydney, we would stop and, no doubt, remember the woman from Meath who spoke to us of a love that was boundless, a union that was indissoluble, and who gave us a momentary glimpse into the mystery at the heart of life.

The Last Two Leaves

ANTHONY J. CHIARAMIDA, MD

On the branch she stays by me
When others all have gone
By reason, fallen, after change
Their season's work all done.

But there, alone, she stays for me
When it was smart to go
October's cold shook weaker souls
Piled so high below

And all together on the ground
They rushed to run away
All together, abandoned hope
One and two and three

And yet the last one isn't last
It mocks both death and time
And holds to life as sure as I
The last leaf on the tree...

The Pediatric Arrest

ANDREA A. PETERSON, MD

We are called to the code, like we are called to all codes during our watch in the hospital. As the senior resident in internal medicine, I am at the helm of the resuscitation team. By now, I have run many codes. They do not scare me; I know what to do. At this moment, however, I am terrified. Tonight it is a girl, 8 years old or so, who is lying unresponsive in the emergency department. I do not treat children. They are small, and they seem fragile and medically mysterious to me. I do not know how to dose their medications properly without looking them up. I worry that there may be many other things about children that I do not know.

I have attended only a few pediatric codes. Usually the child is already improving by the time medicine arrives, and the pediatrics residents no longer need our assistance. We leave, praising the heavens as we go. "Thank goodness," we sigh once out of earshot. "I don't know how they can handle that. There are reasons I chose adult medicine." Tonight, though, this girl is very, very sick, and I will have to stay and help.

The atmosphere in the room is calm and controlled. This is the way it is in codes. Right now, nothing else in the world exists except our attempt to save the life of this one little girl. Everyone works quickly, with precision and coordination. The attending, the senior pediatrics resident, and I stand at the foot of the bed. From here we receive data and suggestions, collaborate, and determine each next step. The medicine team is performing chest compressions. They watch the cardiac monitor and report on the girl's status. The pediatrics residents have unrolled "The Strip," a long, narrow laminated sheet with intricate details about how to properly dose emergency medications for weight and age. The many others present—anesthesiology attendings, medical students, nurses, respiratory technicians—are doing the hands-on work of trying to save this child, who looks so pale and still. Inside the room there is no emotion, just the persistent methodical rhythm of data—discussion—decision, data—discussion—decision. Though I know we worked quickly, in my recollection everything is slow and measured and contained to a three-foot space around a bed, as if elsewhere all time had stopped.

But time has not stopped, not in our room and not in the world outside it. We begin to assemble the girl's story as nurses glean details from her family. It turns out that she is diabetic. Her mother, who is expecting, was hospitalized for a few days because of a complication with her pregnancy and had been discharged just this afternoon. The girl's father had not been around much, so the girl had been in the temporary care of some aunts and uncles. The girl, away from her mother, began to act up, demanding sweets and refusing to take her medicine. The aunts and uncles felt sorry for her and did not know what to do. To appease her, they let her stay up past her bedtime, eat candy, and skip her insulin. The aunts and uncles do not know much about diabetes.

Now this 8-year-old girl is in my room, and she is in florid diabetic ketoacidosis, and she is dying. As I process her heart rhythm, her blood pressure, and her oxygen saturation, I note her blond hair and skinned left knee. I can almost see her climbing a tree, sharing secrets with her best friend, twirling her hair absentmindedly as she gazes out her classroom window rather than at the blackboard. But now her strong, healthy-looking young body is failing.

We have been working for 10 minutes, 30 minutes, an hour. The girl is intubated, ventilated, hydrated. She has been given insulin and bicarbonate. The results from her arterial blood gas return, and despite all our interventions, her pH remains close to 6.0. I am not sure I have ever seen a pH that low in a patient. I say, "We should dialyze her." I know that it is 10 o'clock at night and that it will take another half hour at least to get the dialysis catheter in and the machines set up. But still my eyes turn to the emergency department attending, pleading with her to agree that yes, let's pursue it, there is still hope.

Instead, the attending gently begins to point out that the girl's oxygenation also remains terrible. Her blood pressure is low. Her electrolytes are in severe disarray. She has multiorgan failure, and although we have done everything we could for an hour, nothing has improved. Even if the girl were to survive, her brain has suffered such a prolonged hypoxic and metabolic insult that she would probably never wake up.

I look around the room and can tell that everyone agrees. I ask if anyone has further suggestions about what to do, but in response, there is only a terrible, sad silence. I search the faces of the pediatrics residents, and it is clear that they are already accepting the truth against which my own heart still wants to struggle. I have never seen a child die, not even in medical school, and I almost cannot comprehend a death so preventable. My medical mind can understand it, but the rest of me cannot. We stop the resuscitation. There will be no more trees, no more secrets, no more sleepy daydreams. I walk out of the room slowly and feeling sick. There are reasons I chose adult medicine.

Soon after the girl dies, her pregnant mother arrives. She is brought to her daughter's bedside, where all is still, and voices are low. She begins to cry; soon her sobbing transforms into a wail filled with such profound grief and longing that I think that in all the world this can only be the sound of a mother who has lost her child. The rest of the emergency department is quiet, paying respect to this terrible tragedy. It is as if the universe is acknowledging that nothing is right, nothing is kind, and nothing makes sense.

I sit in the near-dark at the nurses' station filling out the necessary paperwork. I am on call all night, so I will not be able to go home and hold my own 3-month-old daughter until morning. I listen to the sobs of the dead girl's mother, and I too begin to cry and cry.

Homeless

FRANK DAVIDOFF, MD

My mother, Ida, died a few years ago. By itself, her death could hardly be seen as a remarkable event. But the way she died was another matter altogether, because in the week before her death she was quite convinced she was already dead. Here's what happened.

Well along in her 97th year, her body was failing in every way imaginable. The problem list? A virtual textbook of geriatric medicine: cataracts; hearing loss; a small lacunar brainstem stroke (vertigo, diplopia), which had knocked her walking, already shaky, down a notch. Third-degree heart block, pacemaker duly implanted; atrial fibrillation; left ventricular hypertrophy from long-standing hypertension; vasospastic angina. Ischemic colitis, following the block-related bradycardia, which had mercifully resolved; a bleeding pre-pyloric ulcer, the antibiotic treatment for which was, in her view, decidedly worse than the disease. Urinary incontinence (pads, wet sheets, the inevitable recalcitrant bladder infections), osteoarthritis of the knees, impressive leg varicosities, and more than a little dependent edema.

As though this weren't enough, there was the mucous membrane pemphigus that had appeared some 25 years earlier; even on low every-other-day doses the consequent chronic glucocorticoid therapy had slowly melted away her muscle mass, to the point where she was barely able to walk with a walker, or lift a glass to her lips even with both hands. The skin on her legs had become tissue paper: tearing, bleeding, ulcerating—not a pretty sight. Come to think of it, the relevant text here may not be a book on geriatrics; it may be the Book of Job.

But mind and spirit? That was something else entirely. For, as she frequently put it (she was inordinately fond of aphorisms), "The chassis is dented, but the engine is running fine." A marriage and family therapist during the last half of her life, she saw clients practically every day until about a month before the end. This wasn't perhaps so surprising. She was, after all, the person who gave herself roses when she made the honor roll in college because her immigrant parents didn't know American traditions; who got her doctorate in education in her 50s; and who instructed (in writing) that at autopsy, which she wanted performed, her brain should be examined "to identify the source of my *élan vital*."

But as her body increasingly failed her she found it harder and harder to manage at home. At the same time, her need to safeguard her autonomy, always important to her, became something of an obsession. Part-time aides and helpers, a stair elevator, and hand grips in bathrooms and other strategic spots got her by. Over time, however, it became clear to everyone but herself that these arrangements weren't really working, resulting in occasional medical and functional crises. The idea of a full-time live-in companion and, ultimately, moving to an assisted living facility, were rejected, haughtily, out of hand.

And who can blame her? She and my father had built our house, their first (and designed by an architect cousin), in a quiet "bedroom" town in 1940. After my father died, she'd lived there by herself and lovingly maintained it (new roof, paint, wallpaper, and the like) for half of the 60 years she was in it. Its gardens—wildflowers, roses, peonies, irises, not to mention the biggest Franklinia on the eastern seaboard (she claimed)—were her pride and joy. (She knew the Latin names for every plant, shrub, and tree and would happily tell you what they were.) My sisters and I sometimes said to each other that she would literally rather die than move out.

Yet, in her final months even she started talking about moving. This was not every day's decision. Some days, leaving was declared unthinkable; other days, she was unequivocally finished with the house and named the assisted living facility where she wanted to go (she had once been on its Board). Then came the days of increasing somnolence, tachypnea, and cyanosis. And, soon, ambulance, hospital, oxygen, endless questions, chest x-rays, CT scans, lung scans, antibiotics dripping in the vein, and chest tap.

Here the plot thickens. In the depths of that last admission she was truly "out of it" for several days: delirious, babbling, seemingly reliving large chunks of her life, then periods of unresponsiveness. During one long night of delirium, she kept repeating, "Is it easy? Is it hard?" and when, on a hunch, my wife asked, "Ma, are you asking about how hard it is to die?" my mother had said simply, "Yes." Her doctors and we were quite convinced on several occasions that the end had come, but she backed away, somehow, from the precipice. Her respirations and oxygenation improved rather suddenly. A few days later she was again quite alert, although very weak, and managed to make it out of the hospital to a skilled nursing facility not far from her house (she'd also been on the Board of this one).

Sitting with her a day or two later while she ate supper—incredibly slowly—she suddenly paused and asked, very clearly: "Do you mean to tell me I'm still alive? I thought I was dead!"

"Of course you're alive! What were you thinking?"

Silence.

Then someone said: "You know, Ma, what people do to be sure they're alive? They pinch themselves."

She put down her glass, reached over, and very deliberately pinched her wrist. A peculiar expression crossed her face, and she said: "Well, I'll be damned!"

Although we had no reason to doubt her seriousness, things had taken such an unusual turn that we did wonder if she was making some kind of strange joke. But it was not a joke. Over the next several days she made it quite clear that she was not at all certain she was alive. "I was sure you were here at my funeral!" she said at one point. And to the extent she recognized that she was still alive, she wasn't best pleased. "Dying is so hard, and it's so boring! You mean I'm going to have to go through this all over again?" We tried to reassure her that she hadn't died in the first place, but she didn't seem to be really listening. Quite conscious but increasingly distant, she refused all care, quietly stopped eating and drinking, and died in the nursing facility about a week later.

Over the next few months, we pondered what this curious state of mind could possibly have meant. We wondered if it was simply the final stage in her lifelong struggle to confront mortality. We were aware, in that connection, that in her last years, she did what she'd always done when confronted with a new and challenging problem— she had read a book about it. (In this case it was Sherwin Nuland's *How We Die* (1); Chapter One, "The Strangled Heart," was particularly well thumbed.) We wondered if part of her—her true inner self— might actually have "died" during her delirium.

But those explanations seemed doubtful—after all, delirium hardly ever results in people believing they're dead—so we gave up thinking about it. Then not long ago we stumbled on a report of two homeless patients who, although quite alert and coherent, had come to believe they were dead (2). The author, a psychiatrist, suggested that homelessness had ruptured his patients' fragile connections to the world, leading to "the eventual disintegration of their identities and the spiral into existential nothingness." He also pointed out that the state of mind in which a person believes either that they and the world don't exist, or that they are dead, was first described in the medical literature in 1880 by a French psychiatrist named Jules Cotard (3). Cotard's syndrome, which is not common, is a delusional state (*le délire des négations*) primarily associated with severe depression, schizophrenia, and multiple sclerosis. It has also been described, however, following trauma, during extreme hyperthermia or self-starvation (3), after torture (4)—and now, with homelessness.

There's a lot more to homelessness, it seems, than meets the eye. Most of us can't even imagine this "poignant and diffuse" condition, this "absence of belonging, both to a place and with the people settled there" (5), a condition so corrosive that it can shred the sense that you and the world even exist. Is it any wonder that refugee status, and immigration—even moving to a new house—can be so intensely disruptive? Should we be surprised that so many older people are terrified by the idea of moving into a chronic care facility? In this light, my mother's belief she was dead may not really have been a delusion after all. More than likely, she simply came to realize that her crumbling body had, finally and irreversibly, torn her up by the roots, cut her off from a central part of her identity, her home. Although she was well protected, to be sure, from the humiliation and physical misery of living on the street, the existential distress of being homeless was harsh; disruptive enough, it seems, to create a state of mind that violated Descartes' fundamental dictum: *Cogito, ergo sum.*

We'll never really understand why my mother thought she was dead. But at least we know she's no longer suffering the torments of homelessness. Rest in peace, Ida.

REFERENCES

1. **Nuland SB.** How We Die. Reflections on Life's Final Chapter. New York: Knopf; 1993.
2. **Christensen RC.** Dead men walking: reflections on Cotard's syndrome and homelessness. Pharos Alpha Omega Alpha Honor Med Soc. 2005;68:33-4.
3. **Pearn J, Gardner-Thorpe C.** Jules Cotard (1840–1889): his life and the unique syndrome which bears his name. Neurology. 2002;58:1400-3.
4. Break Them Down. Systematic Use of Psychological Torture by US Forces. Washington, DC: Physicians for Human Rights; 2005:55.
5. **Hopper K, Baumohl J.** Redefining the cursed word: a historical interpretation of American homelessness. In: Baumohl J, ed. Homelessness in America. Phoenix: Oryx Press; 1996:3.

Spot(s)

BERNARD ROBINS, MD

The telephone call came from the answering service at noon on a hot Wednesday in July 1957. I had been in practice for about a month and was keeping busy making house calls for doctors on their days off or at night. This call was a request to visit a young man sick with a fever. I drove to the house, and I was met by a 15-year-old boy alone at home. His family was away for the day, and he didn't know how to reach them. He'd been well until early that same morning when he'd developed chills, fever, nausea, and a headache. My exam revealed a temperature of 101, some mild nuchal rigidity, and a few purpuric spots on the extremities that hadn't been present earlier, he reported. Several more appeared as I was examining him. I made a diagnosis of meningococcemia.

What to do? A sick adolescent boy and no parents available. I gave him an intramuscular injection of penicillin and called the hospital. No, they would not accept a contagious patient. I called the county isolation hospital. They wouldn't have a free bed for several hours. While I mulled over the dilemma, a distant memory gripped me so tightly that I thought I was living it in the present.

I had always wanted a dog. My father's illness had destined me to be an only child, and a lonely one. My folks' preoccupation with finances in the face of my father's disability left me searching for affection and companionship, and eventually lead me to the desire—the need—for a dog. I begged and nagged and finally Spot, a fox terrier puppy, entered my life. The quid pro quo was that I would have to take care of him. Spot had been separated from mother and littermates, and I was to be both parent and friend to him.

The next six months were the best. We were an inseparable team. Playing, running, fetching—a joyful duo of boy and dog. One day, when Spot was about 10 months old and I was 10 years old, we decided to go to the park to play "chase the ball." The day was bright, our expectations high, but "first an hour at the piano," Mother had said, adding, "and don't forget to watch the dog."

As I was practicing, I could hear Spot barking outside—his eloquent plea to hurry up. Then I heard the screech of brakes as Spot's barking turned to shrieks of pain. Running outside, I found Spot in the street, down and bleeding. A crowd gathered as I hugged him to me, both of us terrified, confused, and helpless. I looked back toward the house, but no one was visible. After a few interminable minutes, a policeman roared up on his motorcycle. His presence was huge as he approached me and Spot, reached down, and pulled us apart. His expression unchanging, the policeman drew out his pistol and fired into the dog. Spot lurched, twitched once, then no longer moved. As the sound of the pistol shot faded away, so did my hopes. Desperate in my loss, I heard a voice behind me: "This wouldn't have happened if you'd watched the dog." Turning, I could see my mother framed in the window. I covered my flaming ears and fled into the house and to my room.

A vulnerable child, absent parents. My mind abruptly returned to the present. I called the local pharmacy–medical supply house, asking them to deliver—stat—two intravenous infusion sets, 5% dextrose in normal saline, intravenous Solumedrol, and intravenous penicillin. In about 15 minutes it arrived, and I started treatment. The hours went by as I watched the boy's blood pressure slowly fall and the rash become confluent and ecchymotic. At last, the critical condition seemed to be stabilizing. The isolation hospital called to say that a bed would soon be available, and I had the ambulance service transport the patient—with all medications being administered. I followed along and handed the patient over to the infectious disease service. A call that evening to the hospital revealed that he was steadily improving.

The next day, I reported the case during staff rounds and received accolades and applause. My ears turned red. I felt elated and gratified, puffed up but at the same time strangely depressed. The glory was mixed with pain because Spot was with me again. I couldn't help but remember how I'd left him vulnerable and alone. Was one of my motivations to heal born out of the memory of Spot?

First Response

JON O. NEHER, MD

I was driving home from the symphony late one night through the downtown area. The traffic was closely spaced and moving quickly despite the rain and the slick road conditions. I had just passed the last of the downtown high-rises when suddenly a dozen red taillights flashed in front of me. I hit my brakes and was thrown into my safety belt. Traffic came to a full stop for a moment, and then began to inch forward again. In my peripheral vision, I caught sight of a pile of clothing lying in the center lane. At first I thought that it was just some garbage that had come off the back of a truck. But as I rolled slowly past, I developed a sickening feeling in the pit of my stomach. The clothing was not arranged randomly. It was held together in some dimly recognizable order.

I pulled over to the median strip and carefully got out. The October rain was cold against my face. A nightmarish light, created by the headlights of the rapidly congesting traffic, glared off the wet pavement. In my immediate vicinity, vehicles were moving quite slowly, and I was able to weave between them to the object on the pavement.

Lying in front of a black Camaro, in a chaotic tangle of clothing, was a man about 45 years old. He looked like a homeless person, with an unkempt and felted beard, brown teeth, and filthy sweatpants. His two layers of long underwear, plaid wool shirt, and tattered cotton coat were all hoisted up around his armpits, revealing a chest that was ghastly white. There was a single deep laceration across his torso that was not bleeding. I squatted down next to him and checked for the pulse in his neck. Nothing.

A small group of other drivers, including the driver of the black Camaro, gathered around. Familiar protocols flashed into my head. Airway and C-spine control. Breathing. Circulation. But I wasn't in my emergency department. I had no Ambu bag or backboard. My first sense was of being totally unprepared. My second sense was that intervention would probably be futile. But lurking right behind that was a fear for my own safety. Something about the secondhand clothing, the matted hair, and the rotting teeth hinted at the possibility of contagion from hepatitis, tuberculosis, and AIDS. I felt a rapidly rising wave of revulsion. I could not bring myself to put my lips to his.

I stood up and found myself looking into the worried faces of half a dozen concerned citizens. We were all standing in the rain, at night, in the middle of the busiest freeway in the state. Cars continued to pass on all sides, weaving around vehicles pulled off to the sides or just stopped in the middle of the road. A part of me still wanted to attend to the victim, but at that instant, it suddenly seemed more important to be sure that no one else was hurt that night.

"This guy may be here awhile," I said to the driver of the Camaro. "Can I get you to turn on your emergency blinkers and keep this lane blocked?"

"No problem," he said, and headed back to his car. In a moment, the emergency flashers were on.

"Does anyone here have a cell phone?"

"I do," another said, "and I already called 911."

"Good job," I replied. I looked back up the freeway toward the center of the city and could just make out the lights of the county trauma hospital. It had one of the best emergency medical response teams anywhere. They would be here in minutes. I had a flicker of hope for the man lying at my feet. Someone with better experience, equipment, and courage was coming. "Does anyone have flares?" I asked no one in particular.

"Yeah, I do," replied another Samaritan.

"Great. Can you run a line of flares from the back of the Camaro and funnel the traffic past in the right-hand lane? We don't need anyone else to get hit out here. I'm sure we are all practically invisible."

While the flares were set, I surveyed the area. A bridge, so high as to provide little protection from the rain, arched over the freeway where we were standing. Gazing on up the road, I noticed a large Mercedes parked on the shoulder. A woman in eveningwear was standing beside it screaming hysterically. A man was trying to console her. Had the victim walked onto the freeway or fallen from the bridge? Either way, I presumed the Mercedes had hit him. I didn't see any skid marks to indicate that the big car had slowed, but they would have been hard to see under these conditions.

I looked down at the wreckage at my feet. Either accident scenario seemed inevitably fatal. But failure to act could easily become a self-fulfilling prophecy. Was it rationalization that seemed to make the personal risk loom large and the potential for benefit vanishingly small? As if she were my conscience, a woman approached me from the small cadre of onlookers. "Shouldn't we be doing CPR?" she asked.

I didn't have a good answer. "Feel free...," I said lamely. She stared down at the man on the pavement for a long moment. Then she turned and silently walked away into the darkness.

A police car rolled up along the left-hand shoulder of the road. Certainly, I thought, the police would have masks and gloves and would be able to get the rescue breathing going. Their arrival had taken no more than a few minutes. There was still time.

A policeman got out of the squad car, walked over to where our group stood, and bent down to look at the form on the pavement. Then he stood up and addressed us. "I'd like all of you to go over and stand on the shoulder. Please don't leave. We may want to ask you some questions." He ushered us over to the shoulder and then returned to the squad car. The pitiful bundle of wet clothing was now left alone in the middle of the freeway.

I stared in disbelief. The policeman wasn't doing anything! How could he know that the man could not be saved? Was he also afraid of contagion? Was he also repulsed by the dirty clothes and felt hair? Were we both waiting for others to come and take charge?

In less than a minute, the ambulance arrived with a show of sirens and strobe lights. I watched intently as it pulled to a stop on the opposite shoulder, expecting a trauma team to jump out and rush forward with backboard, defibrillator, IV lines, and maybe even a MAST suit. Surely, it was not too late to save him and to save me from my guilt. They could play my role in this tragedy and play it better.

A young woman in a long white coat hopped out of the back of the ambulance and trotted over to where the man lay. She bent down and examined him for a moment, then jogged back to the ambulance. There she retrieved some sort of packet and quickly returned to the middle of the freeway. After she ripped off the tape, the packet unfolded to become a large white sheet that she used to cover the man completely. There was going to be no salvage attempt.

The policeman was out of his car again and looking for potential witnesses. He asked me if I had seen the accident. When I said that I had arrived just seconds afterward but had seen nothing, he told me to leave. The experts had taken over.

I carefully crossed the freeway to get to my car. Shaking the water from my coat, I climbed in and soon gently eased back into traffic. I drove the rest of the way home half-expecting some other madman to dash out of the darkness or perhaps fall out of the sky. The slapping of the windshield wipers punctuated my somber reflections.

I could feel good about having stopped and about having made an effort to protect the crowd. But it was wrenchingly uncomfortable to acknowledge my own ugly bias toward a poor, luckless transient. In a moment of crisis, I had faltered. But I did not falter alone. Every potential rescuer had looked briefly and then simply turned away.

Physics

JOHN J. KEVENEY, MD

It has come to that.
Your life is a rumor
a whisper in a crowded room
an exclamation point in someone else's day
The ending of a path.

The white coats bunch in the corner,
line the walls. Not like before
when there was some procedure to do
something to save, words to say.
They come and leave in a rush

Did the old ones who could do nothing
do this better? Could they be with you
at this passing time. See the light go
feel your presence slide away

Did they know
this was like your beginning
a point in being that is sacred
one of those times when
energy is neither created nor destroyed

An Arctic Moon

JAMES L. GLAZER, MD

"You don't need to worry about my eye," Doc said as he squinted up at me through the bright lights of the trauma bay. "The left one is glass anyway!" A conspiratorial smile spread across his face, compressed and molded by the ill-fitting cervical collar.

Moments earlier, Doc had been brought into the emergency room. Elderly, hard of hearing, and sporting a chart full of comorbidities, he had driven his ATV into the back of a road grader. The piece of heavy machinery rolled backwards, crushing him beneath its wheels. Here in northwestern Alaska there is no pavement, and ATVs are the only way to get around. Doc's family had been trying to get him off his Honda for a year. They had feared that his declining health would lead to an accident such as this.

At first Doc bantered with us as we busily set about surveying his injuries and attempting to stabilize him. After a lifetime in the small community, he was known to all of the nurses and related to more than a few. But his blood pressure, initially borderline, continued to decline despite our attempts at fluid resuscitation. We called for blood, then for albumin. Finally the x-rays came back. The trauma series revealed a badly shattered pelvis. We labored for the rest of the afternoon, running through twelve liters of intravenous fluids and the only four units of type-nonspecific blood in the hospital, in a desperate attempt to make him stable enough to transfer. Then Doc developed disseminated intravascular coagulation. The trauma surgeon, consulting from 600 miles to the south over the phone, was clear in his assessment: "Don't wait to stabilize him. Get him on an airplane now. If he doesn't get to the operating room, he will die. You may still lose him in flight, but traveling is the only chance he's got."

Doc's condition never improved. The MEDEVAC team bundled him up and raced him to the airfield, only to radio 15 minutes later to report that their cabin had suddenly depressurized at 14,000 feet and that they were coming back. Doc was returning to us.

He had developed ventricular fibrillation as soon as the cabin depressurized. The MEDEVAC crew coded him through the return flight and landing. One of my partners met them at the airstrip and saw that there was nothing more we could do. She called the code there, on the tarmac.

A day later I sat with the rest of the medical staff as we went through our code review. "Maybe I should have called the trauma team in Anchorage earlier," one of the physicians said. "If I had transferred him sooner, Doc might have made it." "I could have been more forceful with the lab in asking for blood," a colleague volunteered. We all could have come to help sooner, we finally agreed. Each of us blamed ourselves, in small and large ways, for Doc's death. I sighed and looked down at my hands. What else could we have done better? Could we have saved Doc's life?

Looking around the table at us, the medical director finally spoke. "I have been a part of many cases like this," she said. "This man could not have survived his injuries. We can work to make the system more efficient, but nothing could have changed the outcome. In the end, we can't save everyone."

My partners and I left the room in a somber mood. Though we knew the medical director was right, it was difficult to accept her words. That day I revisited the case often, pausing between patients in clinic to remember each detail of the code. I became more and more certain that Doc couldn't possibly have survived.

Toward the end of the afternoon Doc's family came to the hospital to make the final arrangements.

I have always felt a little strange about seeing family members after the death of their loved one. I worry that on some level the survivors blame me and, if not, that at the very least I must be a reminder of their pain and unhappiness. Mostly, though, I just don't know what to say to them. So when I saw members of Doc's family drifting through the halls that evening I tried to avoid them. But a young woman called me over before I could escape to my work. "Doc was my *tata*, and this is his wife," she said, introducing me to a small elderly lady in a wheelchair. I hesitated, not sure what to do. I was caught.

The seated woman reached out to me. I knelt before her and she took my chin in her hand, pulling my face into her field of vision. "I was in Anchorage when Doc came in," she told me. "I tried to hurry. I felt I had to get home. I knew something was wrong." Mutely, I nodded. She went on, telling me she was too late and that her husband was already dead when her family brought her to the hospital. "Thank you for all that you did, Doctor," she said warmly, giving my chin a squeeze. I hadn't said a word. I watched the family shuffle down the hallway, wheeling their grandmother before them.

Doc's funeral was held in the Friends' Church, a modest structure painted a faded fire-engine red near the center of town. I walked there in silence with a friend, another physician who had supervised much of Doc's care. The church was not difficult to find. In a town as small as this, half of the vehicles were on their way to the church. The other half were already parked in its lot.

The minister, a straight-backed man about 70, with a quiet yet firm voice, gazed out over his people. He wore traditional high mukluks under his business suit. "Doc lived his life a happy man," he began. "He always said you should do the best you can. He loved to mush his dogs. His best day was when they gave him a jersey inscribed with the number 1. It was last year in the sled dog races. They wanted to honor him. He worked hard. He worked on many buildings, on the college in town and the Eskimo World in Barrow. He worked on this church. He pounded many nails when he built it. You might even see the marks where he missed. Sometimes it is hard to pound a nail perfectly. You miss and make a little crescent mark on the wood, like a little moon. The wood is no longer perfect. You marked it with a moon. And that is how you can tell that you have been there. If there were no marks, if Doc had never missed, how could we tell he had ever been here?"

Later, we filtered past Doc's family in a receiving line. I recognized most of the congregation from seeing them as clinic patients in the past few weeks—a consequence of working as a doctor in the Alaskan bush. Last of all, I met Doc's widow sitting flanked by her sisters at the end of a pew.

She took my hand and leaned forward as if to whisper a secret. "I'm sorry," I stammered. Then I paused, not sure where to go or how to explain my disjointed feelings of responsibility and guilt about not having the power to save her husband.

She looked understandingly at me, nodding sadly. "You should always never blame yourself for the things you can't control. Who has never made a mistake? You learn if there is a lesson, otherwise you go on. You will make crescents in your carpentry just as my husband did. How else will you remember who you have touched? How else would they remember you?" Then she held my hand, or I held hers. Neither of us spoke again.

I walked out of the church that evening into a clear, cold night. My breath tinkled as its vapor condensed into ice against the silent backdrop of the Arctic winter. I looked over my shoulder at the church, the light from its windows spilling warmly into the parking lot. Inside, the funeral had given way to a renewing of kinship ties. Mothers visited with each other while their husbands told each other lies about the fall's hunt. As I turned to begin my walk home, the sky caught my eye. There, against a brilliant backdrop of Arctic stars, waxed a new crescent moon.

Empty Pockets

KEVAN PICKREL, MD

Many of the experiences in our work we smooth and shape in the retelling like pebbles being polished by the tides. Some are more valuable for their sharp edges and the pain and lesson they bring by holding them tight.

I spent part of my residency training at a city Veterans Hospital. Overnight call meant perpetual motion punctuated by frantic episodes of critical care. On this night we had done well, and by the time the first "code arrest" sounded overhead we all had managed to keep our heads above the tide. We arrived to the medical intensive care unit, wearing the authority our white coats gave us, to a bedside now ringed by staff. A trach collar had come loose and the trach itself unseated, but all had been corrected. Sorry about the run.

A curtain separated beds in this area of the intensive care unit, and each curtain had been pulled when the code was called. I lingered to one side, planning to stay long enough to see the collar retied. I was jostled by some movement at the adjacent bedside. The next time, it was followed by an arm. My name was shouted, then I was pulled by my coat sleeve through the curtain to the next bed. The patient, a woman aged 36, had been admitted by one of the teams earlier that day. Chest pain, they said. The bedside monitor began to bleat and flash. Her blood pressure was falling with each systole, and her cardiac tracing was taking on the jagged, wide, rugged contour that meant we were in for a difficult time.

Her husband and two young daughters, 8 and 3 years old, were led away from the bedside as the intubation tray was being opened. Quickly intubated, compressions made obtaining central access more difficult, but I placed an internal jugular line hoping things would go well enough that it might be used for a Swan-Ganz catheter. Compressions, fluids, advanced cardiac life support protocols ... all the while cardiac tracing into dysrhythmia. Occasionally, the monitor would only stare blankly asystole, across its screen. And the blood pressure. Boluses and drips and fluid, nothing would move the blood pressure. *She was only 36.* I reached deeper into algorithms, knowing the next vial off the code cart would run the answer into her collapsing circulation. The answer that would also push away the pain growing in my own stomach. I believe I tried everything, and trusted each new intervention would be the one. None of them changed the course. Boluses, drips, compressions, bagged breaths, time, her heart finally stopped. *She was only 36.* I silently asked myself, "Why?" A nurse touched my arm and said the two words whose weight made my next breath difficult and whose grip was tight around the pain in my stomach: "The family."

They had been taken to the waiting room. It was pale blue and the row of lights indicated the soda machine was still empty. My throat was dry. The youngest daughter sat on Dad's lap looking at pictures in an outdoors magazine. The older sat watching her hands rest in her lap. Her husband's eyes lifted to me and met mine. I didn't, couldn't, say a word. I took in the breath to begin, and he knew. The words never meant quite enough. "All we could ..." They seemed small, like a string of toy boats against a stormy sea. "Her heart ..." I only had to say the words; the family would have to live with them. "So sorry ..."

He turned back toward his daughters, a single father, and they lifted their eyes to his. As he drew the breath to begin, his eldest daughter knew. Suddenly all alone, she stood and ran toward us standing at the door. Dad bent toward her, but she got past him to me.

Tears an unbroken line down her face, she took hold of my coat pocket. She said words that made six years of medical school, residency, and late nights too numerous wither. "Give mommy more medicine. She'll get better, but you have to give her more medicine, please." I couldn't breathe. I had no words, no gesture. Her dad bent to her, but she wouldn't let go of my pocket. He nodded to me, indicating I should go, and as I did the pocket she held tore.

I drove home, tears making the road focus and unfocus, replaying it all to find the why or how. Ruptured ventricular wall? Aneurysm? Pulmonary embolus? I stopped when I realized it didn't matter. I went home to my wife. As she stood silently watching, I took off my doctor's coat and put it in the trash. Later I could explain. All I could say now was, "That one doesn't work anymore."

The Cardplayers

GEORGE N. BRAMAN, MD

Over the houses of the dead my shadow passes.

Paul Valéry, *Le Cimitière Marin*

I see four cardplayers among the stones
Intent upon their game, they play their hand
Indifferent to departed souls or bones—
The graves look on impassively≠ and bland.
I see this image from a passing train,
Just one of many a successive scene—
It hovers like a tune or old refrain
and lingers like the daggers of a dream.
Like a playful Caravaggio print
On a whitewashed canvas planned with skill
The cardplayers in melancholy tint
Play out their game, though oblivious still
To the names etched on the indifferent stones,
Their forfeit lives, their scattered whitewashed bones.

A Walk on the Beach

DAVID S. PISETSKY, MD, PhD

In August of each year, I take a two-week vacation with my family, wanting to get as far away as possible from the hospital where I'm the rheumatology division chief. We rent a cottage on the beach, and I do my best to avoid any thoughts of medicine, patients, sickness, or death.

Although I claim I do nothing on vacation, my day is actually full. I swim in the surf, I walk on the beach, and I fish for spot and pompano. The high point is in the evening when I sit on the porch, drink Jack Daniel's, and savor the warm moist air that sweeps in from the sea.

At the end of my vacation, I return to the hospital looking tan and fit. My mind is clear and my spirits are boosted, at least for a while. This year, however, my plans for rest went awry when, on the Monday of my second week on vacation, I decided to take a walk on the beach.

It was late afternoon. The sky was silver-blue and the heat was thick. Above me gulls soared and the sun shined molten white. As I walked, thinking about which seafood restaurant to go to that night, I heard the piercing sound of a siren and the blare of a horn. A fire truck and an ambulance rushed by in the direction of a fishing pier that the hurricanes had reduced to a skeleton of blackened pylons and planks. After the fire truck and the ambulance came two police cars. About a half mile from the pier, I saw groups of people looking at the water where a pontoon boat was navigating figure eights. I picked up my pace and began jogging.

I came up to a woman whose eyes were riveted on the pier. The woman's back was red from sunburn.

"What's going on?" I asked.

"A man is missing," she said, squinting into the sun.

"What happened?"

"Not sure. The man was in the water when his family drove off for a while. When they got back, he was gone but his boogie board was on the beach. They're hoping he's taking a walk but he may have drowned."

I continued jogging to the pier and heard another siren. As I approached the pier, I saw a boy running frantically along the beach. He looked about 10 years old. His thin legs churned as he ran along the beach, stopping every few seconds, jumping up and down to get a better view of the water. It was the missing man's son, I decided.

When he got near the rescue boat, the little boy hollered across the waves to the men in the boat, heard something, and then ran up to one of the houses. The house was flying an American flag that slapped in the wind. "They didn't see anything yet," the little boy, breathing hard, shouted to two women on the porch. He then ran back to the beach.

I climbed up onto a dune so I was close to the porch where the two women stood in floral bathing suits. I didn't need a family tree to figure out who they were. Clearly, these were two sisters, and one of them was the wife of the missing man. They had long curly hair that streamed in the wind. They clutched each other and their eyes were tight.

"They have to find him," one of the women said as she pressed her head hard against her sister's chest.

I would like to say that I hung around because I am a doctor and might have been needed for a rescue, but, at this point in my career, my skills in emergency medicine are trifling. I was just another spectator, gripped by the drama.

An older woman then came out of the house. This was the man's mother. She wore thick eyeglasses and a pink housedress. She went over to the two younger women and they all clasped each other.

By now, over 100 people were along the beach, standing silently on the dunes. We all looked at the sea as the rescue boat bounced in the surf and weaved around the remains of the pier.

A woman with a stethoscope around her neck came out of the house. She called to the older woman and together they went back inside. Then I saw two EMTs push a gurney onto the street. On the gurney was an old man with white hair. This was the missing man's father. He had on an oxygen mask. His hands covered his eyes and his body shook. I was ready to offer the old man help, but this looked like heartbreak, not a heart attack, and there was nothing I could do. It was almost 6 o'clock, and I had promised to take my family to dinner. I was late, so I left the scene, agitated, anxious to know what happened next. As I ran homeward, up the beach, I saw a Coast Guard boat speed toward the pier, then three helicopters, hammering the air and making my body throb.

By the time I returned to our cottage, I was flushed and sweating heavily. For a moment, I thought about going into the ocean to cool off, but I was repelled by the thought that I would smack into a cold, waterlogged body washing up on shore.

That night at dinner, everything about the meal seemed tired and dreary as I talked about the events on the beach.

"You have to be *so* careful in the water," I said to my daughter.

The late news didn't have a story about the rescue so I had to wait until the next morning to learn the outcome. At the market where I buy shrimp for bait, I learned that the missing man had been found dead by a fisherman that night. The man had died boogie boarding, his neck apparently snapped when he was flipped by a crashing wave. He was only 36 years old, the girl at the checkout register said.

Later that day, I took a walk in the opposite direction from the pier, not wanting to come upon the dead man's family as they packed up the cottage, loading the roof racks on their Chevrolets and minivans for the ride back to Ohio or Pennsylvania or wherever. What an awful trip they had ahead, I thought to myself, wondering how they would get the dead man's body home.

Because of the accident, I told my daughter to stay close to shore, warning her about fierce currents. My conversations with my wife—normally about books or movies—kept returning to the man who drowned.

"What a way to go," my wife said as we walked on the wet sand of low tide. "That poor family. Their lives are ruined."

Over the next few days, I toyed with the idea of leaving on Friday or Saturday instead of on Sunday, wanting to get a jump on the mounds of work that I knew awaited me at the hospital. We decided to stay, but I didn't go swimming again.

On Sunday, driving home while listening to a golden oldies station, I knew that I had wanted to leave early because a dead man haunted the beach. Seeking respite in a hospital may seem strange, but in my office near the clinic, I feel protected and secure. At work, wearing a white coat, my guard is up. My defenses are arrayed. On vacation, wearing sunglasses and a T-shirt, I am an ordinary person, subject to ordinary feelings when terrible things happen.

In the hospital, a place of incredible loss, we try to keep death tame. We confine it to wards and hide it behind curtains. These acts of control are an illusion. Under the sky and near the sea, death flies free.

It has been more than a month since I returned from the beach. I will soon start my stint as a ward attending and undoubtedly will have to talk to a family about a patient whose condition has worsened. In the narrowed and reddened eyes of the family, I will see the expected reactions—grief, fear, longing—but because of what happened this August, I will also see something else.

I will see a vigil on the beach. I will see three women clutching each other as they rock in the rushing wind. I will see an old man overcome as he lies strapped on a gurney in the searing sun.

Most of all, I will see a little boy, a little boy who runs up and down the beach in a desperate search, who hopes and hopes against hope, yearning so much for one more chance to see the joyful face of his living father.

The Finished Product

BONNIE SALOMON, MD

Don't think the clocks will stop, the planets freeze in place.
Don't boast of celestial standstill. (God doesn't press a pause
    button.)
Don't pretend your passing will be the colossus of the ages,
The eighth wonder, the end of an era. It will be a nuisance.
From the nursing home, off to paramedics—
At the ER, the nurses and doctors sigh, "Shift change—let's get
    her upstairs,"
Slap high fives as you force your last cough.
Orderlies take you to the morgue, with unfeeling care,
Hurry to dispose before lunchbreak. Mounds of paperwork
Cause a disgruntled intern to pout. Forms fill with details.
The who-what-why-where-and-how of you. Unbecoming becomes
a busy burst, someone else's trouble. Be not proud of death:
Mysteries do not concern the bureaucrats.

Precious Cargo

KATHIE KADRI, MD, PharmD

Infatuation. A feeling of such intensity that I recall being startled by it, and my life was not the same thereafter. It was 11 December 1979, just past dawn. He was across the room from me, in an incubator because of a difficult birth. He lay on his side, looking toward me, pensive, calm, with incredible, large dark eyes. The most beautiful newborn I had ever seen. I fell deeply in love. I would not again experience such feelings for any child. Daniel was the first in many ways: first child of my brother, whose wife was my dear friend; first grandson of my father; first nephew for me. He was born into a farming family, the great-great grandson of a Montana homesteader. The farm would be his if he so chose. My husband, my father, and I lived next door to the new family, and we all reveled in the child. Every milestone was pure delight. His intelligence was evident early as his vocabulary blossomed. My favorite memory of his early childhood recalls his mother reading a book. She was lying on the floor, propped on her elbows, with crossed ankles in the air. She loved to read. Her son was beside her, with his own book, imitating her pose exactly. He was less than 2 years old. They were inseparable.

Separation. I stopped after work to get him from the wedding reception his mother was attending, so he could be in bed on time. His

mother's parting words were, "Be sure to buckle him into his car seat."
He was precious cargo. She would drive home later, alone. A drunk
driver would cross the centerline and take her life, at age 24, pregnant
with her second child. Her son was 2 years and 9 months of age. He
continued to ask for her for a long, long time. He wondered where she
was and why she was not coming home. Deserted, abandoned, rejected—how else could a child that age feel? There was no way for
him to comprehend why she left and would not come back. Our hearts
were broken: my brother's, the child's, my father's, my husband's, and
my own. We tried to fill the void in his life during that first long, dark
winter of her absence. We all tried. We healed slowly, or so it seemed.
I was the primary woman in his life then, but I could not replace his
mother.

Replacement. His father remarried. A baby brother and then a sister
would join the family. I moved away. Daniel was a quiet child, unde-
manding, in contrast to his half siblings. His large dark eyes remained
breathtaking, and I often wondered what deep thoughts they hid. It
was difficult to get him to share his feelings. He was so unlike his ex-
troverted father, but his mother had been quiet and introspective, so
perhaps he had her nature. I watched him grow from a distance, seeing
him once or twice yearly. He seemed content, but I worried. Was he
getting enough love and attention? Was his stepmother treating him
well? What scars from the loss of his mother were hidden from me?
His father's second marriage ended when Daniel was in his early teens,
another loss for him.

Repair. Stability came from his father, his grandfather, and from
the farm itself. He developed a sly sense of humor and a quick wit,
which revealed his deep intelligence. His grin and his laughter were
infectious. He learned from his father how to hunt, fish, and ride. He
adored his cousins and great-uncles with whom he hunted every fall.
He treasured the outdoors. He worked daily with his grandfather on
the farm, gaining wisdom from the elder, the elder gaining strength
from the growing boy. He earned a brown belt in karate and won
awards. His father remarried again, a new stepmother that Daniel admired for her hard work on the farm, side by side with his father, and

for her shared love of hunting and the outdoors. It was to her that he
took his mending. He graduated from high school and started college.
But he seemed unhappy to me. His stepmother thought he should
move out on his own, but I felt he was not ready. We went to dinner,
and I told him I worried about him. I thought he might feel deserted
because of the women who had moved in and out of his life. I asked
about his relationship with his stepmother. "Talk to me," I said. He
assured me that all was well, and so I believed him.

Confidence. He joined the National Guard, won awards for marks-
manship, and received promotions. He moved into the hired hand's
quarters on the farm, which he customized in comical and touching
ways. A 5-foot metal flower leaned against a wall. A bison skull wore
dark glasses and a camoflauge baseball cap. An orange recliner and a
green lamp were salvaged from his grandfather's old house. Pink
flamingos gazed from a shelf. A baseball cap collection included some
of his grandfather's that he donned playfully and laughed at with
friends, but then lovingly replaced back with the others. Small magnetic screwdrivers formed an awning around the range hood. The refrigerator joked, *It's not premarital sex if you don't plan to get married,* but
it also proudly displayed a certificate for completing jury duty and a
ribbon earned for judging a contest. He grinned as he showed me his
treasures. He had found a college major he liked. He played paintball
and practical jokes with his friends. He fought forest fires with the
National Guard and was thrilled with the new skills he'd gained. I
spent a week on the farm in the summer of 2000, in his proximity. He
had acquired an ease with himself, and with those around him, that I
had not previously seen. He was physically mature, tall and muscular,
seemingly invincible. I loved to hug him and feel his strength. I set
aside my long-standing uneasiness about his well-being. I made him
the primary beneficiary in my will. He would inherit my farmland
and his mother's ring that I wear. He was my surrogate son.

Rejection. He was late for chores on an October morning. His
grandfather went to the hired hand's quarters to fetch him, so they
could start them together as they often did. He found him there, in a
pool of blood on the kitchen floor, with a handgun nearby.

Death by suicide is the most profound rejection, of self, of family, of life. I care for patients nearing the end of their lives. Cancer or organ failure ravages them, yet they fight for every minute, willing to undergo any invasion, to prolong life. How could this child, in robust health, intentionally terminate a life so full of potential, when so many would do anything to live? How is it possible that we who nurtured him could not sense the anguish that allowed the deliberation of loading a handgun, placing it to his temple, and the final volitional act of pulling the trigger? I have searched his 20 years in my mind, over and over. What signs did I miss? We quizzed each other, his friends, his teachers, his girlfriend. We replayed his recent behavior in our collective thoughts. Had he been quieter, less involved, losing his temper, missing class, avoiding work, not seeing friends, or using drugs? The answer was no, to all. On the contrary, he was applying for a summer internship, fixing his car, making plans for the future. Only a recent disagreement with his girlfriend stood out, but he had left her a note the night he died: "You are worth fighting for and I won't give up." Then why did he?

Pain. Shock, denial, anger, guilt, pain, unbearable pain. Why, a thousand times why, did this happen? I can comprehend this suicide only as an impulsive act, yet I did not know Daniel to be an impulsive person. I know with certainty that this was unplanned, because he would never have wanted the grandfather that he loved so dearly to find him as he did. Was it an "I'll show her" act from a wounded heart in a young relationship? Does it really matter? He made a choice, whether a split-second decision or one pondered for years. The consequence is the same. He is gone from us forever. Yet, it does matter, because I cannot bear to think of this child as feeling unloved and in despair, not this child. I cannot stand the pain of thinking that he did not know his worth to us. He was precious cargo. His loss causes a sadness within me that feels infinite and inconsolable. Watching his father and grandfather wrestle with their pain and guilt adds much to the weight of my suffering.

Cleansing. His body was gone when I arrived, but his blood was not. Two large pools, so much blood that it took almost an hour to wipe it away. His father and I cleaned it from the kitchen floor. His grandfather could not bear to enter the house. I needed to do that duty; I wanted to have his blood on my hands. It was all that remained of his physical being. The cleansing of his blood seemed to be the final gift, the last labor of love I could give to my lost child. Now the enormity of our loss settles in with the darkness of winter. I wonder about the months ahead, and whether my elderly father will live long enough to recover from the shock of finding his grandson dead on the floor by his own hand. I fear the effect of my nephew's choice on his siblings, his cousins, his girlfriend, and his best friend, who in his eulogy said he had lost a brother and a soul mate. I wonder how I will rebuild my faith in the future. My husband is my source of strength, and he has the soul of a poet. He tells me to explore this void, the place this child occupied in my life. He says to move to the edge, peer deep within and gaze across, navigate the distance around, acknowledge this place, respect this place, but do not fall in and be lost to it.

The Cancer Cells Sum Up

RAE VARCOE, MA, MB, ChB

I am startled by the blue beauty
of the cancer cell
it is bound only
by its neighbour's intimacy
integrating itself softly
like an exotic alien
into the unresisting tissues
of its owner

here, it insinuates
into the artery's intima
stretching its luxurious surface
along the endothelium
to reach the cut margin
where its compatriot
has already set sail
like a pirate
moving to claim territory
in the wider shores of the lungs

this elegant mosaic
each regular azure tile
annealed to its neighbour
is interrupted only
by the exuberance
of mitotic figures
announcing new divisions
heralding multiplication
adding up to extinction

A Good Pair of Hands

BHUVANA CHANDRA, MD

He greeted me as he always did, hands folded weakly together in the gesture of respect that is ubiquitous in India. *Namaste:* "I bow to the Divine in you." He could barely lift his head from the thin pillow, and his emaciated arms trembled uncontrollably from the effort of opposing his palms as I approached bed 6, row 2, in a second-floor ward of the Government General Hospital in Madras. Embarrassment heated my face at the reverence that lit up his tired eyes and rekindled, for the tiniest moment, the fading sparks of what had once been the natural élan of a 12-year-old boy. To him, I was God—weren't all doctors? His faith humbled me at the same time that it angered me. Did he not know, could he not see that I—a newly graduated physician, still unsure of my right to be called "Doctor"—could not cure him? The typhoid bacillus that scavenged his small intestine and poisoned his blood also eluded the antibiotics pouring into his veins. I am *not* God, I screamed silently, even as I sat by his bed and gently disengaged his clasped hands, careful not to grimace at the putrid stench from his abdominal abscess, smell of my failure. The skin of his palms reminded me of a dried-up riverbed, with arid furrows crisscrossing from the wrist to the joints of his fingers. Calluses like rough pebbles dotted the outer edges of his hands. His fingers quivered in my grasp.

Tiny red beads crowned some of the fingertips where drops of blood had been pricked out by his caregivers, to reappear as complete blood counts on the pages of his hospital chart.

For four weeks now, he had been my patient. My predecessor had relinquished him to me, signing off on his chart with an expression that was at once sad and relieved. For four weeks, I alternately pleaded with and raged against the invincible intruder that silently ravaged the boy's once-sturdy body, whittling away flesh and muscle until the boy looked like an ad for Oxfam. He neither moaned nor cried, not even when his gut burst and made pain his constant companion. Surgery would have banished this unwelcome visitor, but the boy was too malnourished for the knife. I smuggled in bunches of fruit—fat bananas and juice-heavy oranges—and slices of coarse white bread dipped in broth, determined to plump up his frame, to win the war against wasting. His hands had become bony echoes of their once-sinewy selves, and he struggled to clasp them around the peeled fruit and hold the bread steady between his thumb and his fingers. We played a game: He would tell me about the harvest waiting to be plucked by his hands alone when he returned home, and I would compliment him on how well he held the fruit within his palms.

Those hands had once firmly pulled on cattle reins as he plowed the small acre of soil adjacent to his grandfather's hut. He moved in circles with the cattle from dawn to dusk, occasionally curling his hands around a bamboo stick and prodding the cows when they tired. The same hands had planted tiny seedlings of rice and lentil seeds in the hard soil, watering them with tenderness, anxiously unfurling newborn spears to check for insects and mites. They hauled hay for the cattle to feed on and milked their swollen udders dry each morning before the sun bloomed and collected their waste to use for fuel. His agile fingers shaped the freshly steaming dung into round, flattened cakes, which he then laid in long, horizontal rows on the thatched roof of the hut so that the noon sun could bake them into stone-hard tinder. His small frame gave no clue to the strength in his capable hands, a strength that served him well when it was time to fill the glazed earthenware jars and aluminum drums in the kitchen with water from the well in the backyard. The heavy braided rope that coiled around the pulley above the well slipped easily through his hardened palms as he carefully lowered the metal bucket deep into the blackness below. The bucket's return journey, the water as heavy as concrete, might have caused rope burns in another's hands, yet he managed the burden with ease, proud that hardly any water sloshed out.

His grandfather fed him when he returned to the hut at the end of each hot and tiring day, plying him with *dhal* and rice and milk and an extra piece of mango secretly saved from his own earlier meal. He then rolled out the straw mat for the boy to sleep on, the one with the extra padding. His grandson was all that stood between him and starvation; *he* was the boy's all. Since the boy fell ill, the old man had been floundering, unable to till the land on his own, lost without the youngster's able hands. He visited him once a week and stayed the night; the rickshaw *wallah* charged three rupees one way, and it was a long journey for a 70-year-old man frail with worry about the future.

Now, as I prepared to change the soaking dressings on his grandson's abscess, the old man, silent as always, reached forward from where he sat rigidly on the steel chair to the right of the boy's head and covered the child's hands with his own. Carefully peeling away each dank piece of yellowed gauze, I watched as gnarled fingers, dark brown and crooked with age and toil and arthritis, stroked with infinite care a pair of hands aged before their time, hands that should have held schoolbooks and tossed rubber balls and spun wooden tops and colored glass marbles on the hard-baked ground in the company of children. The boy winced as I started unwrapping the final stained layer. It caught on a bleeding edge of the abscess and, rather than risk further bleeding, I decided to cut it away.

Even simple tools like scissors were scarce in an overburdened state hospital in India. I opened a pack of razor blades and, pulling one out, cautiously sheared the rank wrapping, bit by bit, until I had reached the final rancid shred adhering to the wound. At that precise moment, the tug of the blade on the cloth produced such a sharp shift in the inflamed tissue that the boy spasmed in pain, jerking his hands out from under his grandfather's and involuntarily pushing up at my wrist. The blade sliced through my left middle finger before any of us realized what had happened.

He was inconsolable. Long after I reassured him that it was a superficial nick, long after I had stanched the minor bleeding and cheerfully bandaged my finger in front of him, even long after he lay with a fresh white dressing on a clean bed, the boy cried quietly. His grandfather and I sat on either side of his narrow pallet, and as the ward grew hushed and shadowy and nurses with starched caps hurried softly by, we placed our hands on each other's and over the boy's and listened to the sorrows of life that seep so naturally and simply through a hospital's sterile walls and regulation steel beds. A young boy wilting before the harvest, an old man left alone to reap.

He died the next morning. I placed the banana I had brought for him on the metal bedside table and looked across his shrunken body at the old man, sitting stiffly in the metal chair. A faint effluvium of pus lingered like a blessing in the air. He stared at his grandson's peaceful face for the longest time, then said, "He had a good pair of hands."

I know the boy would have liked that.

Cleansing

NATALIE A. MARIANO, MD

She lay still, so frail and quiet you would think that she had already died. But when I walked into her bedroom and spoke her name, her eyes opened and lit up. Her life was in her smile.

Her husband stood at the foot of the bed, relating the events of the past several days. She ate a few bites of scrambled egg this morning. He gave her drops of medicine through a straw. She was too weak to get out of bed, but he changed her position every two hours, just as the visiting nurse had shown him. She had spells of coughing that frightened him.

She had no complaints. That did not surprise me. In the 12 years I had cared for her, she very rarely complained, and when she did she was self-conscious and apologetic. She had accepted her diagnosis bravely. When we realized that her cancer could not be cured, she fretted more for her husband's future than for her own. They had been married for almost 50 years. Their children were grown and lived out of state. Who would take care of her husband after she was gone?

I examined her much more closely than was necessary. She would die soon. The small bedsore on her back would not affect the quality of her last days. But her husband had paid attention to every detail of her care, and I knew that I must do the same. She was clean and diapered and smelled like lilac powder. I knew that it was he who kept her that way. The sheets on her bed were spotless and white. Her pink cotton nightgown had been freshly laundered and interwove a glimpse of color between her sheets and her pale skin. A soft, puffy quilt lay neatly across the bed. Her medications were lined up in rows on the bedside table with a fresh glass of apple juice and a bright box of tissues.

I told her it looked as if she had a very attentive nurse, as if someone was taking good care of her. She looked at her husband, smiled, and agreed. But he would not take credit. "She's the one who's always taken care of me."

He was tall and thin. He had once been a construction worker. He had little to do with the cooking and cleaning and the rearing of four children. He went out to work early each day, came home, changed his clothes, and ate dinner. Each night, she carefully shook out his clothes and washed them. She had no way of knowing that the asbestos fibers in his work clothes could pose a danger to her health. Nor could he have known that caring for him could ultimately play a role in her death. Years later, when we discussed her disease together, I never shared my suspicions with them. As I stood with him at her bedside, I wondered whether they had ever guessed. I prayed that they hadn't.

We quietly left the room, and he led me to a linen closet. He reached under a stack of sheets and brought out a framed photograph of a beautiful young woman. "This is what I took with me to the war, and this is what got me home again." His eyes could look only briefly at the picture before they filled with tears he would not let fall. He quickly slid the picture under the stack of clean linens and went back to care for his wife.

Death with Dignity:
A Case Study

WALTER J. KADE, MD

I voted twice against legislative measures in Oregon that would allow physician-assisted suicide. Within months after the Death with Dignity Act became law, I received a call from the parents of a patient of mine requesting that I assist their daughter in her suicide.

My patient was then only 29 years old, but she seemed much older and wiser. I had diagnosed her non-Hodgkin lymphoma almost 10 years earlier. She was not only bright but also intensely perceptive and private. With a thin, angled countenance, thick, dark hair, and rich, introspective eyes, she was a startlingly handsome young woman. For several years she had lived independently from her parents in a smaller community adjoining ours.

During one of her periodic visits home a decade ago, my patient's father became concerned about her frail appearance and asked that I see her. I was not concerned after the first evaluation and attributed her minimal complaints to youthful fatigue. Only at her father's urging did I make a second, detailed evaluation. I will never forget my shock when I viewed her chest x-ray to find the mediastinum bulging

Editors Note: The family of the patient described here has given its permission to publish this study. At the family's request, however, the author agreed that his real name would not be used. Walter J. Kade is a pseudonym.

into both hemithoraces. The course of her disease during the subsequent years was relentless. Conventional therapy and bone marrow transplantation ultimately failed. Alternative medicine failed. Experimental protocols failed.

She became slowly, but quite assuredly, terminally ill. Still, she managed to lead an amazingly active, full life. She continued work on an advanced college degree and nearly finished it. She became engaged to a young man who shared her values and perspectives, such that the two of them seemed almost to merge into one. She maintained her talents in the arts, writing short stories, pursuing the theater, appreciating the beauty of the world in ways that few seem capable of.

As she became progressively sicker, she moved home to the love and care of her family. Although she now was routinely seen by oncologists, we maintained our relationship, and I continued to be her primary physician and friend.

Thus, it was with some surprise that I learned of my patient's wishes. Although I knew her illness was terminal, her life seemed to me to be far from terminal, and in most respects quite remarkable. She was engaged to be married; she still pursued many meaningful activities; and she had a devoted and invested family. She did not seem to manifest any of the characteristics that I considered to constitute intolerable suffering. Although she had become physically wasted and required help with most activities, she had no pain, maintained an adequate appetite, and was no longer bothered by the night sweats that had plagued her in other times. Why would she want to end her life? Was her suffering so great?

She had certainly had times of great suffering during the past years: constant pain, unpredictable and wrenching night sweats, anorexia that made days pass without sustenance, protracted nausea and vomiting. But that time of extreme physical suffering had abated. And yet, what I learned was that her disease continued on its inexorable course, more silently now, but gradually and uncompromisingly robbing my patient of her life. Her cachexia had become striking. She was incapable of living the full and independent life that she cherished, that had defined her. As the weeks and months passed, her spirit, that unwavering and tenacious hold on and love for life, had begun to slip away. I struggled to understand her suffering, a suffering as much of mind and soul as of body. Without the physical suffering that I, as a doctor, could more readily identify, I was unable to accept its severity. My intellect rejected participation in the suicide request.

I had no doubts about my vote against physician-assisted suicide and my support for a mandate to protect the public from the risk of seeking death for the wrong reasons. I still think that decision is correct for the public. But my soul nagged at me, for although I believe in protection of the public, I also believe in patient autonomy. I support individuals' rights to make their own informed decisions, whatever their reasons, as long as they are capable of making them and their decisions are legal. I believe that physicians are engaged in a service profession and are "called" to serve their patients. With my intellect and my soul thus engaged in unresolvable debate, I sought out the counsel of a dear friend and wise mentor and laid forth my conflict. He stated simply, "I certainly want to be able to make *my* personal end-of-life decisions." And so, I accepted my new role in helping my patient in her suicide with no inkling of the road that lay ahead.

As the law requires, I visited her the day after she made the request to review the prerequisites and to begin the mandatory 2-week waiting period. She met the prerequisites: terminal illness with less than 6 months to live, the absence of depression, and acting of her own free will. As I joined her and her family at their home, I readily acknowledged that I had no experience in this unfamiliar role. We discussed the requirements: completing advanced directives, obliging open communication among family members, and planning for a detailed discussion of the skills needed to prepare for and fulfill the act itself.

Two weeks passed—only 14 days on the calendar, and yet my lifetime as a physician seemed to replay. What did this new responsibility mean to my patient, to me as a physician? I assuaged my concern by reassuring myself that my patient needed the control over her destiny that having a lethal amount of secobarbital at her command would afford her. I convinced myself that if she were only given the ability to control her life, she would be unlikely to act on it.

At the end of the waiting period, I entered a phase of this journey that I never realized would be as emotionally devastating as it became. I had no colleagues experienced in physician-assisted suicide to whom I could turn for advice, for clues about obstacles or how to handle difficult moments. I read the well-written handbook, *The Oregon Death with Dignity Act: A Guidebook for Health Care Providers* (1), which outlined several points that I had to master to prepare my patient.

As I sat with my patient, her fiancé, and her family that next day, I felt my control unravel as we began to discuss the explicit instructions for preparing the lethal medicine for its ingestion. Ninety 100-mg secobarbital capsules were to be supplied. The patient or her family had to prepare them by opening each one and emptying the powder into a container. Because the powder is acrid, the instructions noted that it should be mixed in a medium that would make it palatable, perhaps in a favorite dessert or liqueur. My patient was to take an antiemetic 1 hour before the planned ingestion to reduce the risk for vomiting and aspiration. She was to make all farewells before ingesting the medication, lest she become too drowsy to complete the task. For the same reason, she was to consume the entire dose within a minute or less if possible.

I lost my composure several times during that hour. Why did I have such trouble giving those instructions, instructions required by the law? I now understand. I was teaching my patient how to end her life. That was my trouble.

My patient and I had now fulfilled all our legal obligations. It took another three days before the medication was available. A pharmacist, who was made unknown to me, dispensed the prescription. I picked it up not at the pharmacy but at an administrative office at the hospital to ensure anonymity all around. The instructions read: *Take as needed.*

When I arrived at my patient's home that evening, I again reassured myself that my patient needed this medication as a way of controlling what might become uncontrollable if she felt her autonomy slipping away, that the secobarbital would sit on the shelf, out of sight and almost out of mind.

She and her fiancé had just returned from three days at their special retreat, to which they had traveled many times before. They returned looking fresh and united. As I gazed at the two of them I was reassured that, indeed, control was the focus of this request.

While I was reviewing the instructions again, as the protocol required, my patient interrupted me and asked, "Excuse me, are you saying that I have to take all of these?" There was not a hint of anxiety or indecision in her voice. There was complete understanding, anticipation, almost exhilaration. She was fully engaged in the discourse, in the planning.

I began to lose my composure again, but as I prepared to take my leave, I somehow managed to say, "I respect you and your decision, whatever it may be. You have the right and complete support of your family and me in determining your own outcome. If you decide not to proceed with this, please know that I am available in any manner you wish. Should you choose to proceed, I am available to your family in any manner they may wish." Although the law allows the physician to be in attendance during the implementation phase of the act, it is not required. Her family asked that I not be present, and I said my good-byes.

That evening was a nightmare for me. I had observed my patient while she received her medication. She had shown determination, positive emotion, almost joy as she listened intently to my reiteration of the instructions. I was certain now that she would act on the opportunity, and my intellect and my soul re-engaged in battle. Was my role as physician now expanding into executioner? What was so difficult about this? I had helped many patients die by withholding life support and even by withdrawing it. What was different here? What about my original premise that this was not right for the population at large? And if I felt that way, why then should it be right for the individual? I recognized only later that my patient's goal was to be released from a life that had robbed her of her independence and dignity; at the same time, my goal was to retain a foothold in a life that was now challenged by a "calling" I did not choose to hear.

Morning came with no disruption of my sleep. I rose thankful that at least she had not acted on her opportunity this last night. How wrong I was! When I checked my beeper for messages, I noted an unanswered page at 1:00 A.M. My answering machine also had a message from my patient's father. Why had I not heard either call? To this day I do not know, but my sleep had been uninterrupted. As soon as I gathered my thoughts, I called my patient's home. Her father answered and said that he had called earlier to tell me of their daughter's death within an hour of her eating the applesauce laced with secobarbital. I blurted out my apology for not being available as I had promised, stumbled over my condolences, and asked to speak to her mother. She came to the phone, thanked me for my participation, and added, "In preparing her ingestion, I gave my daughter the most important gift I could give, and the most difficult one I could give."

Now, months after the experience, I still reflect on it daily. Some issues I have resolved, others remain unanswered. I have since visited my patient's family and fiancé. They all remain most grateful for my participation in my patient's suicide. We had developed a closeness, a union through this event that holds us together still; in fact, so much so that they invited me to become a member of their family. I accepted. My mind is more settled and comfortable with my role in her suicide. I am now confident that I made the right decision for her. She had the right to choose, and the Oregon statute allowed her to act on her decision. Her family and her fiancé also believe that strongly. They were willing to displace their own need to have her with them with her need to be gone. I must do the same; and I have also redefined intolerable suffering. I now believe that it may occur in ways quite different from those that we as physicians normally consider and that intolerable suffering is best defined by the patient. My patient was suffering at the core of her being without agonizing pain, anorexia, or night sweats. She had become increasingly dependent on others for virtually all activities. Her dignity, her self-esteem had been stripped away. The vitality of her being had passed. Yes, her life, as she defined it, had become futile. Finally, I have also accepted that my emotional turmoil in great part reflected my entrance into uncharted territory for physicians. Although we have accepted our roles as comforters in end-of-life care, we have not struggled with or found solutions to active roles in aiding patients in accomplishing their deaths. I am grateful for the great disruption in my emotional stability that this experience precipitated. This act should never be easy, never routine. It should be among the most difficult and disquieting acts we embark upon.

REFERENCE

1. **Haley K, Lee M, eds.** The Oregon Death with Dignity Act: A Guidebook for Health Care Providers. Portland: Center for Ethics in Health Care, Oregon Health Sciences University; 1998.

Pronouncing

BRENDAN M. REILLY, MD

Many years ago, when I was just starting out, I worked in a small New England town where local law stated that the newly deceased were not duly deceased until pronounced by a licensed physician. Legally, the undertaker couldn't take over—you weren't really dead—until a doctor said so.

At first, this sounded harmless enough, even quaintly appealing, a vestige of simpler times when doctors really were gatekeepers, ushering lifeless folks out of the world and delivering new ones into it. But that whimsy dissipated soon. My nights on call, preoccupied plenty with the living, brought frequent "requests" to pronounce the dead— now, tonight, it wasn't "decent" to wait until morning. Whether the call came from the local nursing home or from a distraught spouse suddenly alone deep in the New Hampshire woods, I was expected to drop whatever I was doing, travel to wherever the recently departed had recently departed, and pronounce the passing as officially passed. This seemed to me an inefficient use of my time. After one especially well-traveled night on call I expressed this opinion to the local undertaker, who seemed friendly enough (and remarkably well rested) but who said simply, "That's the way we've always done it in these parts, doc."

In retrospect, this wasn't all bad. When the deceased person or family member was my own patient, it felt right for me to be there. But more often than not, the corpse was that of a total stranger who, like me, had been called unexpectedly to an unfamiliar place with an uncertain welcome. On those occasions, I felt like a cop or a mortician must feel, my words to the family hollow and perfunctory, my presence an invasion of their space and a waste of my time.

And so it happened, halfway through that first year in practice, that I responded none too cordially to a call late one Saturday night from the sister of a man I didn't know who had just died across the river in Vermont at the end of a long dirt road well known for its impassability in winter and washouts in spring. She said Charlie had been a patient of Dr. B. (whom I knew to be a fine diabetologist) and that his sugar had ruined his kidneys and circulation years ago. She sounded flat and matter-of-fact, and I probably sounded the same when I said curtly that I'd get there when I could, that I was busy. (I wasn't.) She started to say something about the Lord and eternity and not to rush, but I hung up before she finished.

I checked my black bag before setting out. Tonight, I saw I was well stocked—epinephrine, penicillin, incision and drainage kits, even an endotracheal tube—but I had run out of death certificates. That about says it all, I thought. I would pick some up at the hospital. It was on my way and, as the lady had said, no need to rush.

The emergency department was hopping, a code and a car crash. The head nurse suppressed a condescending smile as she handed me a fresh stack of coroner's papers. Hey, her eyes twinkled, we've all got a job to do. Then she spun away to assist in the trauma room, where two teenage boys were trying hard to die. Bending over one, a neurosurgeon paused momentarily while the nurse reported the blood alcohol levels, then resumed drilling a hole into the kid's skull. On my way out, families milled in the waiting room, hugging and pacing. A woman with red puffy eyes, cigarette in one hand and a sleeping baby in the other, saw my doctor bag and shouted out to me from across the room, questioning. Everyone stopped, the whole room collapsing into me, a black hole. "I'm sorry," was all I could think to say, "I don't know anything."

The highway into Vermont, well-lighted and smooth, turned to dark and dirt as I began the slow climb into the hills of the back country. Rising, like searchlights on the ocean floor, my high beams swept the black moonless night. Rocks and pebbles pinged the rusty underside of my old Volkswagen, rollicking in the rutted road. In the dark, the dashboard glowed yellow and red and green, blinking like the city night, like the night of my first call to the autopsy theater in medical school. I had stood huddled by the window high above the streets of New York, all alone except for that hulking shape draped on the diener's table, waiting for the pathology resident to arrive, watching the great city far below as its staggered traffic lights rolled up First Avenue from the Battery to Harlem and back again, waves of red then green then yellow then red again, the tides of Manhattan. She was my first encounter with death still warm, that old lady with blue hair, her eyes wide open, her mouth agape, clearly surprised by something. After we opened her up and emptied her out, I knew I would never be the same again either. Tonight, in the hills of Vermont, all of that seemed very long ago.

The dirt road ended abruptly at the top of a rise. Even in the dark I could see or sense somehow the broad breezy expanse of high open meadow surrounding the grand rambling farmhouse and its many large outbuildings. Looking back now, knowing what I know today about this place—its pastures and corrals stretching to the horizon, copses of white birch bending in the wind, century-old beech and maple on fire in the fall, million-dollar views a hundred miles to the east and west—it is easy to feel naive or stupid about what happened that night at Charlie's house. But this was 25 years ago, before the boom, before Montana and Virginia and Vermont made the real estate section of the Sunday *New York Times*, before Charlie's place and the rest of God's country were sold to the stars and the traders and Ted Turner. And so I will tell you what I saw that night and how it strikes me now. But I may never know what really happened.

The house was lit brightly from within, as if a grand party were in progress. Its penumbra of yellow light leeched out into the surrounding fields, which, at the edge of darkness, seemed endless. I didn't dwell on the magnificence of the property because I was so surprised by the youth of the woman who greeted me and introduced herself as Charlie's sister. No older than 30, Carol looked like most young farm women I'd met: no makeup or pretense, an old sweater and jeans, the stiffly graceful gait of a rodeo rider in her prime. She seemed to measure me with her gaze, decided something, then thanked me for coming.

She led me through a series of 200-year-old rooms with low ceilings, original beams, and wide pine floors covered with antique Persian rugs and English hutches. We came to an enormous living room where four men sat guffawing on stuffed sofas around a blazing hearth and a coffee table covered with beer bottles. They looked to be in their 30s, beefy and bearded like well-fed woodsmen, rednecks roistering. Three of them didn't acknowledge my arrival at all, but a fourth lifted his chin in my direction, drunkenly waved a thumb toward a grand staircase behind him, and said dismissively, "He's thataway, Bud." Then, to Carol: "How 'bout some refills, Hon'?" She said nothing and led me upstairs.

Charlie seemed small, almost childlike, laid out in the massive four-poster bed that occupied one corner of the huge master bedroom. Against the white sheets, he looked the palest shade of pasty blue, mottled and cold, unmistakably dead yet undeniably young. He had had diabetes since age 9, Carol said, and was always sick with one thing or another. He had never married.

"Not much of a life," Carol said softly. "But he never complained. When our folks passed a few years ago, he moved into their room here and tried to help run the farm, but he was in and out of the hospital all the time and never could get along with Jack—my husband, you just met him—not that other folks can either."

She started to say more, but her eyes filled. She put her trembling hand to her mouth and swallowed hard. She patted her lips, as if her fingers could free her voice. She began to sob silently, her shoulders shaking. Then she waved her hands, more at him than me, apologizing. I thought I understood. She left the room.

Alone, I did the drill. Apneic. Unreactive midpoint pupils. No audible heart sounds. A few small ecchymotic areas over the abdomen and upper thighs, insulin injection sites. No femoral pulse, just ... what? The slightest flicker at my fingertips. The beating of my own heart? I pushed down more forcefully to obliterate my own digital pulse. Now nothing. I tried again. Once more the faintest movement, deep in his groin. And then, again, nothing. I stepped back, looked hard at his sad lifeless face, then cursed out loud my wishful thinking, my need to help, my desire to win. Perhaps for those reasons—and suddenly grateful that Carol had left the room—I dug into my black bag, flipped open a bolus syringe of D50, felt deep into his femoral triangle again (not a hint of life), and plunged the needle just medial to my fingertips. Feeling like a fool, I emptied the barrel into his groin and glanced up at his face, absurdly hoping for a wince, a sign. Nothing.

I sat down by the side of his bed and waited, whether to confirm the futility of what I'd just done or for some other reason I can't remember. All around the room lay mementos of Charlie's family and the grand homestead they had occupied for hundreds of years: scores of photographs in fine antique frames; daguerreotypes of lean, mustachioed men in Union blue and prim grim women in bonnets on horseback; an oil painting of Ethan Allen dated 1763; ornate sabers crossed at the hilt above a small plaque that read simply "Iroquois 1684." One more recent photo held my gaze. In a high meadow surrounded by blazing fall foliage, Charlie and Carol stood with their parents, none of them smiling but all holding hands, the picture of family solidarity and understated Yankee pride. I thought of my own little kids and wondered whether they would understand what was important to their parents, whether they would carry on any of it after we were gone. As Charlie apparently had tried to do.

I went downstairs. Carol was waiting for me. I offered my condolences, but I don't think she heard me. Behind her, the men around the fireplace were even louder and rowdier than before. One of them, short and powerfully built, had taken off his shirt and was spraying beer at the others and all around the living room.

Carol led me away from them—they paid me no attention—to a table at the far corner of the room where I sat with her and began to fill out the death certificate. She succinctly provided the information I needed—his age (36), next of kin (herself), other survivors (none)—all the while watching me with a strange intensity, searching my face as if looking for an answer to some unspoken question, straining to read upside down what I wrote. I thought I had seen this behavior before, when I had to tell a young mother that her two-year-old daughter was dead, drowned in the pond behind her house while she answered the telephone inside. And so I just assumed that I couldn't answer Carol's unspoken questions. Besides, the whole scene gave me the willies: The three other men were now spraying beer back at the first man, his bare hairy belly slathered with foam, all of them hooting and hollering.

Hurriedly, I finished the paperwork, grimacing (as I always did) when required to fill in the *cause of death* for a patient I'd never seen alive: "cardiac arrest" (always a safe bet) *due to* "possible myocardial in-farction" (who could argue?) *as a consequence of* "long-standing diabetes mellitus" (ah, science!). Thus pronounced, Charlie could now meet his Maker, or at least his undertaker.

I rose to leave. As I extended my hand to Carol, she avoided my gaze and, for just a moment, I felt a twinge of guilt, aware that I could have done more, for her if not for Charlie. But then I became aware of what can only be described as a deafening silence, the complete and instantaneous loss of all sound in a room that had been so rackety and loud just a split second before. Carol began to rise slowly to her feet, her face suddenly drained of all color, transfixed by something behind me. As I turned to look, one of the men muttered in a deep trembling voice, "Jesus Christ!" and there, at the foot of the stairs, stood Charlie.

Pale as a ghost, arms extended and eyes half-shut, this apparition seemed to float into the room. It drifted silently toward the hearth where the four men sat, now suddenly sober, bug-eyed. The log fire crackled and leapt, as if stoked by the specter's approach. Recoiling, the men stiffened, pushing back deeper into their seats, unable to move or look away. Now the specter stood before them, oblivious to their presence, as if it occupied some dimension disconnected from our own. It began to lick its lips and shake its gruesome head from side to side: No. No. No.

Suddenly, with unexpected swiftness, it reached down toward one of the men. He gasped. For an instant it hesitated, cocking its ear as if listening to some distant sound. Then it reached down again, grabbed a fresh bottle of beer from the table, popped it open, and drank greedily, all of it in one ravenous chug. Then it leaned back and belched, a prolonged guttural gaseous eruption so gross, so uninhibited, so natural that it seemed to expel forcefully from the room the otherworldly atmosphere. No ghost, Charlie blinked, looked about, and seemed to see us all for the first time. In a hoarse, indignant voice he said to no one in particular, "Jeez, I'm starvin'. Where's the fuckin' food at?"

Pandemonium. The men roared, gleeful, shouting, slamming their fists down on the table, punching each other playfully about the arms and chest, swigging their beers and toasting Charlie, who stood quietly before them, their straight man. They pushed two more beers into his hands, threw a big bag of potato chips at him, and began to sing some swaggering song I didn't know, something about lads and battles and bottles of beer. In the uproar I didn't think to look at Carol, but the next thing I knew I was standing next to Charlie, taking his pulse, introducing myself, beginning to explain, and then she was there too, pale as a ghost herself, in a cold sweat, touching his arm and stroking his hair but staring at me, her face contorted in anger.

"*What is this?*" she hissed.

Charlie, preoccupied, reached for the bag of potato chips.

"*What is this?*" she said again, louder, to me.

"Chips," Charlie answered.

Working Against the Grain

DAVID P. STEENSMA, MD

I paused under the carved lintel that crowned the doorway of his battered clapboard farmhouse. Despite the sanction of the Hippocratic Oath (*Into whatever houses I enter, I will go into them for the benefit of the sick ...*), I remain uncomfortable when entering my patients' homes, especially when there is little to offer beyond the dubious benefit of my presence. The probing intimacies of routine medical practice don't bother me much anymore, but home visits still seem a deeper invasion of privacy—like sitting abruptly on the corner of an occupied hospital bed, or eavesdropping on an unguarded telephone conversation while reading a chart outside a room.

But that night's visit felt different. Neither my patient nor I knew yet that he was dying, and neither of us knew that the same disease that would take his life would soon touch me, too. For more than a year, the farm's owner had been urging me to visit his expansive wood shop, his passion and pride; it was the only thing I had ever known him to boast about. After months of delays and indefinite plans, and a long drive through gathering dusk on increasingly rough and lonely two-lane roads, I had finally arrived. I reassured myself that I was there by his special invitation and found the courage to ring his doorbell.

Though he was not quite 60 years old, he was my oldest patient, and over time, he had become a friend. In the first few weeks of my medical internship, I inherited his care from a departed resident. Back then, we had little to do together beyond keeping a watchful eye on his blood pressure. Yet, his clinic visits were always a pleasure, because there were so many more interesting matters that we found to talk about: the sturdy cradle he was racing to finish before his youngest daughter went into labor; a magnificent lot of old-growth white pine he bought from a marine salvage company, dredged at unbelievable expense from the muck beneath Lake Superior; or the medicinal herbs growing in his wood lot that he sold to cover his bills at the lumberyard. After three years and the end of my residency, we parted company. I moved on to a hematology–oncology fellowship and assumed I would not see him again. But a few months later, he surprised me by showing up in my new clinic, now with a deep melanoma on his leg. The invitations to visit the shop began soon after his surgery.

The door into his home opened. I followed his cherub-faced wife across the length of the house, toward the pulsing throb of heavy machinery. From conversations in the clinic, I had expected his living areas to be filled with impressive hand-hewn sideboards or perhaps cabinetry built for the ages. Instead, the farmhouse was cheaply furnished with obviously factory-made pieces.

His wife spied my disappointed glances and smiled knowingly, wistfully: She would have loved to keep some of his work, but he gave all the best pieces to other people. Before she knew he was this way, back when their love was new, she was hurt by his apparent insensitivity. She would become attached to an immaculately rendered highboy or a sturdy whatnot, only to return from the grocer's one afternoon to find a newly empty corner in the living room. Inevitably, she would learn that he had given her treasure to an acquaintance who was newly divorced, or to a family burned out by a house fire that he had read about in the town paper, or to the widow of a favorite high school teacher long since forgotten by other students. Now, after 30 years together, she knew him infinitely better, and her frustration had turned to immense pride, especially because he gave these gifts anonymously, without fanfare, so that almost no one knew his secret.

Before leaving me at the doorway of his noisy domain, she showed me a utility room stacked high with finished furniture awaiting future local sorrows. Her face tightened as she told me how he had been working lately at a tireless, breakneck pace. She did not understand this unprecedented day-and-night effort, and it had begun to cause her worry. Despite this relentless productivity, the quality of his work was stunning. The chipless dadoes and rock-solid mortise and tenon joints, all cut and fitted with true craftsman's skill, appeared likely to survive us all by centuries. I appreciated for the first time the surprising capability of his thick limbs and of the rough hands that I had unwittingly examined so many times. His gifted extremities were repeatedly dismissed in my clinic notes with nothing more than a terse declaration of their continuing freedom from clubbing, cyanosis, and edema. Eyes see only what the mind knows.

The door to his wood shop opened stiffly, reluctantly. As I pushed my way in, I penetrated drifting clouds of sawdust, the heavy sweetness of machine oil, and the sharp odor of fresh varnish. I found my friend bent over a lathe, slowly turning a post that looked progressively more like a table leg as I watched him work. When he finally noticed me, he powered down the thundering machinery and pulled off his goggles.

He showed me around the empire of tools that he had gathered over the decades. Bulky, cryptic machinery rested in orderly right angles on the shop floor. As in a great factory, the plan was carefully arranged to follow his workflow. I had never seen a collection of clamps as vast as that hanging from my friend's pegboards; he insisted that woodworkers, like surgeons, can never have too many clamps.

We then passed a dark storage room with a cheap plywood doorway, a room that he claimed was an embarrassment, his "Chamber of Heroic Failures." He seemed so sheepish about entering that I hardly dared pass through the door behind him. His voice dropped as he looked at the scattered wood fragments and described to me his first fumbling steps into woodworking, after he had returned shell-shocked from Vietnam. Horrified by what he had been ordered to do in the Mekong Delta and bewildered by the awkward reception he had received upon coming home, the sureties of the wood shop became his refuge and sole comfort. Unemployed, he spoke little to anyone for more than six months, seeking daily absolution for the fires visited on the jungles of Southeast Asia among the sparks that flew from his borrowed sander, all the while trying desperately, futilely, to forget. Since those painful early days, he had saved all of his flawed pieces—never consciously intending them as *memento mori*, but insisting that he was keeping them just in case he ever needed to salvage some irregular bit of wood for another project. Eventually, he found that he could no longer bring himself to break any of them apart. From the thickness of the cobwebs in this room of mistakes, it was clear to me that there were few recent additions.

Most of his failures came when he tried to work against the grain. When he took extra care to follow the natural inclination of the wood, mishaps became much rarer. I had just returned from a conference in Tuscany, and I offered him the consolation that even the greatest sculptors sometimes misread their raw material: Michelangelo abandoned the *Florentine Pietà* after Christ's leg cracked irreparably, even though the figure of Joseph of Arimathea was a self-portrait. My friend seemed unconvinced, looked at me sternly, and countered that skill *matters*—reminding me that Michelangelo carved the great marble block that became *David* after several lesser sculptors had failed, overwhelmed by the magnitude of the problems it presented. He wondered if I would offer the same comforting platitudes to the surgeon who resected his melanoma, if the surgeon had accidentally sliced a nerve or clipped an artery.

We quickly moved out of the shadowy room and toward the comfort of the kitchen door. After a cup of green tea ("Melanoma cells hate it," he assured me) and toast with blackcap jam—taken at a kitchen table ordered from the Sears catalog—I took my leave.

A few months later, his melanoma returned. Now it was in his lungs, beyond the skill of even the most visionary surgical sculptor. I enrolled him in an experimental protocol of a new vaccine, uncertain if we were following the grain or cutting across it. At his next visit, he developed patchy vitiligo; was this a good omen? He joked that I was stripping away his tough old oak stain and replacing it with aspen— lighter, but more fragile, too. His scans remained stable. Our unspoken worry was that rot was advancing secretly somewhere beneath the surface.

Finally, the veneer cracked. His wife called me late one night, crying bitterly. I learned that he had torn himself away from the wood shop long enough to take a fishing trip on a remote lake with his son-in-law. Suddenly, without warning, her husband had slumped over in the boat, unresponsive. After a harrowing journey back to civilization, he was brought to our medical center by helicopter. Neurosurgeons dampened his intracranial bleeding but could do nothing for the ebony sawdust of recurrent melanoma scattered across the folds of his brain.

I walked through the door of the neurosurgical critical care unit to where my patient lay dying. I sat silently next to his wife, her eyes now dry. Together we watched the neurosurgery resident's spidery fingers adjust a metal fixture on the intracranial pressure monitoring device bolted into his skull. The room was warm, and the dried blood around the bolts mingled with the sweat from his brow. Despite the heaviness of this moment, I smiled inwardly at the connoisseur's delight my patient would have taken in the complex clamps pinning the bulky monitoring device to his head, imagining how eager his thick fingers would have been to test its resilience.

His wife now understood why he had been laboring with such inhuman energy since his melanoma was first found—why his wood shop had, for the second time in his life, become a reason for living, rather than simply a treasured hobby. But I did not know the fire driving his work until I was surprised by my own malignant tumor the following year, not until I struggled to return immediately to work despite postoperative narcotic haze and plenty of sensible advice to the contrary. I did not truly understand what drove my patient until I was overwhelmed by the need to sublimate the first real taste of my own mortality, even as I perversely enjoyed the irony of immediately following board certification in oncology with a personal diagnosis of cancer, as if the regulators' seal and authority were not quite enough. I did not understand the cold purpose behind my friend's frenzied carpentry until I found myself racing madly around my laboratory, trying to finish off all the half-done projects that did not also seem half-baked, able to ignore the blood on my clothes, yet stopped abruptly by the clever clamping mechanism of a thermocycler lid that I had been using daily, unseeingly, for years. And I did not understand his need to throw himself wholeheartedly into the work that he knew would be his lasting legacy until I let myself imagine how my young children would remember me, and realized just how quickly it would be before they were the only ones who did remember.

The next day I returned to the neurosurgical unit, but he was gone. I received an invitation to the funeral home, but sent a letter of condolence and flowers instead. That was one doorway too far for me to follow—for now.

Last Hope

H.J. VAN PEENEN, MD

Heart, the capital city, when informed
that death was at the palace gates,
hauled his standard down.

He could no longer count on his defenders,
those lounging bodyguards, lungs, kidneys, eyes,
already conniving to remain alive.

They'd take the victor's shilling if they could,
a chance to live in someone else's shell.
That hope he thought as hopeless as his own
but still he said, "Enjoy yourselves, go out,
be free and young. I wish I, too, could live
the metaphor of love, say *heart*
as though it were a passion, not disease.
There will be dancing in the streets tonight.
Go! May young girls at very brink of life,
but needing lungs or kidneys, give you
the virgin joy of an unbroken heart."

But did those gay seducers of the night
succeed? Ah no, at dawn
the Black Marias filled and now
the firing squads line up. The brain's
already gone, the others barely worth
a transplant surgeon's being called from sleep.

Their hour has come but still the organs pray
for miracles, the fabled midnight call.
Who knows? Perhaps a sleepless governor
will take an interest in a kidney tired
from seventy years of metabolic work,
an eye whose cornea has grown opaque,
a lung burned by a lifetime's oxygen.

The wild canary (or as i die)

MICHAEL C. PETERSON, MD

i cough and smother, my
grown daughter cried when that young
doctor said "malignant effusion . . ." and morphine,
morphine makes me whirl and sick, and i

twirl back through pretty oil pastels to
dandelions, my sundress, our tetter-totter, and
a hot slide on bare tan legs, but

in my chest—something's angry, and i
choke and it pushes, a
bird flicked past my window now i think, and i

saw a little bright wild canary once when i
played with my sister in
the creek and we splashed and squealed, but

now tears work out me—not sad, and i
hear—not feel, my throat croak and gurgle, and
don't breathe, and
life was beautiful as i die

OxyContin

ART VAN ZEE, MD

It might have been easier
if OxyContin swallowed the mountains,
  and took
the promises of tens of thousands
  of young lives,
Slowly, like ever-encroaching kudzu.
Instead,
it engulfed us,
gently as napalm
would a school-yard

Mama said
As hard as it was to bury Papa
after the top fell
in the mine up Caney Creek,
it was harder yet
to find Sis that morning
cold and blue,
with a needle stuck up her arm.

OxyContin

Top of her class,
with nothing but promise ahead
until hi-jacked by
the torment of needle and spoon.

Hospitals,
Health Systems,
Contentions

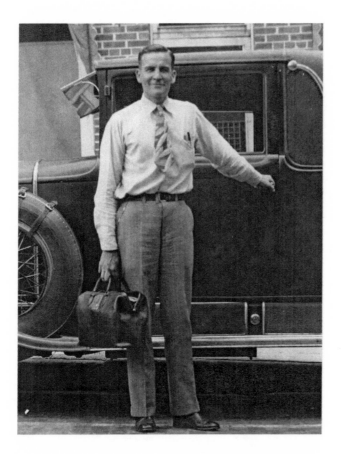

Dark Rounds

FAITH T. FITZGERALD, MD

It's 5 A.M. and I have just finished rounds on my busy general inpatient service. I have done a history and physical exam on eighteen patients—of whom ten were new admissions—on eight different, geographically separate nursing units on five floors. I am tired, but the day has not really begun. I must dictate my notes; go over yesterday's correspondence; answer phone calls from the East Coast (the Midwest and West Coast will have to wait until "working hours"); attend morning report, teaching rounds, and various meetings and conferences; and see outpatients, students, and faculty. By 3 P.M., I will be a mental fungus.

Being a teaching attending in an academic medical center has changed since I was a house officer 30 years ago. My attendings would come in three days a week, sit with us in a small room for an hour and a half, listen to the presentation, and then (perhaps having shaken hands with the patient, though just as often never having seen them) discuss the pathophysiology, biochemistry, differential diagnosis, and therapeutics of the disorder (which the patient might or might not have) of greatest interest to the attending. Care of the patients was almost entirely in the hands of the housestaff, and it frightens me, in retrospect, to think of the decisions we made alone.

Now, on a university internal medicine service, my team of resident, two interns, a senior student on clerkship, and two to three third-year students admits patients three days out of five. Each patient must have a history and a physical exam done personally by the attending, and the work must be extensively documented in a formulaic but periodically inexplicably mutated style acceptable to the third-party payers and the federal government. A daily follow-up exam and note on each "old" patient are also required. Inpatient length of stay is significantly shorter; technological diagnoses are considerably more detailed; and, depending on how one constructs it, teaching rounds often less resemble the archetypical faculty discussions than they do faculty functioning as a senior resident on work rounds.

My hospital has a schedule not unlike that of most academic teaching centers. The housestaff sees their patients before morning report. At 8:30, we meet for an hour at morning report, then, at least three days a week, we proceed to teaching rounds for two hours. The afternoons are left to work, new admissions, and discharges. The teaching attending, who is often assigned for a three-week period, may also need to meet his or her other obligations throughout the period of the attending stint. There are no longer the weekends to catch up on paperwork, because patient care does not stop on weekends.

Perhaps most disturbing to me as an attending is the frequent inability to even find the patients, far less their charts. The hospital is a hive of activity during the day. Patients are taken away from their rooms for diagnostic studies, visited by consultants, or moved from room to room to accommodate other patients. Just tracking them down is a major effort, let alone spending time with them to listen to their history and do their physical exams in anything remotely resembling an environment suited for the interchange of intimate details between patient and physician.

"Teaching" rounds have become the presentation to the attendings of the facts of all the cases, which leaves little time for any discussion other than of the immediate pragmatic necessities for care and rapid discharge under the pressure of utilization review. When I observe the other teams, as well as my own, it seems that the flow of information no longer moves from attending to student. Now it moves mostly from housestaff to attending, so that he or she can write billable notes. I could not remember the names or faces of my patients, much less the increasingly severe and complex multiple symptoms and findings they presented. It was particularly difficult when I would have ten patients in follow-up and ten new patients to evaluate in a single day.

One day, I do not know why, perhaps on another errand or by some whim, I got myself up out of bed and came into the hospital very early in the morning—about 3 o'clock. I discovered a place not that unlike the predawn hospital of 30 years ago. The charts were all in their racks, the nurses were eager to tell you what was going on with your patients, and the patients were in their beds. Housestaff on cross-cover occasionally rushed by, but seldom had time to chat. I thought that the only differences between this place and hospitals that I remembered from my youth were the ubiquity of a blaring television over the foot of every comatose or confused patient's bed and the computer terminal from which laboratory results could be readily obtained—but only at night, when there is not a line of house officers and nurses waiting to use the modem.

I found out who my newly admitted patients were and visited them one by one. Having recently come in, they were dreadfully ill and did not seem to mind being visited by the attending early in the morning. Their rooms were relatively quiet once I turned off the television set, and I could sit at the bedside and listen to a history, do a physical exam (actually hearing murmurs and bruits because the decibel level was low enough to allow for such sensory data to penetrate), and compare my findings with those of the housestaff admission notes. I was delighted to find that I could still discover things housestaff did not know and so augment their work. I could easily write notes in the charts because the charts were there. I genuinely enjoyed the feeling that, during teaching rounds later that same morning, I knew exactly which patients I wanted to take my housestaff to see to demonstrate physical findings, to illuminate a piece of history, to model interactions, or to make inquiry at patient bedside of their impressions. Some patients told me, in a variety of ways, that they wanted us to come by as a team, both for their therapeutic comfort and because of their desire to participate in teaching. I was prepared to discuss the issues surrounding the patients, because I had already met all of them. Most of all, I did not feel rushed. I had seen the patients, I had written the notes, and now the two hours of teaching rounds could be pure teaching.

And so I began to come in during every attending stint in the darkness before—way before—the dawn and more wonders appeared. The nurses appreciated the time and the colleagueship and could tell me things that I otherwise would never had known about both the patients and themselves. Their generosity of spirit, their true concern for patients, and their professional expertise became much more evident than it had been to me in the more frenzied daytime. I was able to teach them, and they were able to teach me. I also had time to speak to families, particularly those of the seriously ill. They deeply appreciated an uninterrupted discussion about their loved one; again, a rarity during the daytime. Far from resenting my early visits, the sentient "old" patients asked me to be absolutely sure to wake them when I came, as they had much to tell me. I was able to dictate the findings of the complete history and physical exam very early in the morning, and I had that record, both of new patients and follow-ups, in the chart by that same afternoon. I felt once again as if I were making a contribution to patient care, rather than serving in a secretarial function for billing purposes. I actually began to think that what I said might make a difference, not just in the generation of clinical revenue, but because people might read my work-ups and get ideas from them. In short, write-ups became more enjoyable and less rote documentation for faceless bureaucrats to use to decide whether or not I was a cheat.

Other advantages became clear later. I began to be seen as virtuous by my colleagues and by those other services whose staff habitually worked nights: surgeons, emergency department physicians, on-call housestaff. I was one of them and thus to be respected. Best of all, by late afternoon, people knew that I was functioning poorly and often excused me from committee meetings and the other ancillary delights of academic medicine. After all, by 3 o'clock in the afternoon, I had often already been working for 15 hours (minus a nap for an hour or two).

Not everyone can work this schedule, obviously. Some are constitutionally unable—a matter of biorhythms, I think. Others have families who would protest, and justly. It is not with a recommendation that all physicians follow suit that I write this piece, but rather to let those teaching physicians who are unhappy, frustrated, rushed, and harried in the modern academic environment know there is a quieter place, an older place, a more fulfilling place—the subdued hospital in the dark of night.

The Cost of Medicine

SHYAM K. BHAT, MD

It is obvious that the patient is dying. She is 92 years old with "multiple medical problems"—so many that my tired intern mind can barely list them on morning rounds. "History of metastatic colon cancer, diabetes, advanced dementia, congestive heart failure ..." But the family wants everything done—so we do our job efficiently and thoroughly. The attending physician recommends an MRI to clarify the diagnosis of the patient's sudden limb weakness, and I write the order down, then initial it. It feels routine now, this mundane ordering of expensive tests with no questions asked about cost. No more do I feel the sense of wonder and amazement that suffused me when I first started working as a physician in the United States. Like "Medical Disneyland"—as many diagnostic and therapeutic rides as you want. And no lines in *this* amusement park, Sir! So I ordered them all, the MRIs, the CTs, the PET scans—this was larger-than-life medicine.

But for some reason today, as I order the scan and look into the hazy eyes of this 92-year-old woman with a dying body that all these thousands of dollars will not save, I think back to the boy.

*　　　*　　　*

While a medical student in India, I was on call one night in the ER (or "casualty," as it is known in India), asleep soundly in a room that I was sharing with the intern, when we were awakened by loud knocking on the door. The government hospital could not afford pagers, so the system of choice was Ramappa, the orderly, who was sent to wake up physicians whenever there was an admission. The method was a bit alarming, especially at two in the morning, but it was foolproof—there was no "But my pager didn't go off!" I woke up with my face and scalp itching. A few mosquitoes had made their way through little rents in the mosquito net and now in the dim light I could see them hovering around, replete and sluggish.

"What is it?" the intern asks sleepily.

"One boy has come to Casualty, Doctor. He feels sick and wants medicine." Ramappa had a talent for giving us no information at all yet managing to sound like he was imparting details that were clinically crucial.

We go to Casualty where a boy sits in the corner wearing a ragged cotton shirt a few sizes too big and blue shorts, the color beaten out of them. His bony legs are dry and scarred and his bare feet do not reach the ground as he sits on the stone bench. His hair is wispy brown, his eyes sad, and his belly protrudes below prominent ribs. This small front room is used as a waiting room but also, when things are busy, as an examination room or sometimes even for minor surgical procedures. There is no door—it was never designed for one with its wide archways and open windows—and the smell of disinfectant is not as strong here in the cool night air. Moths fuss around the bright lamp on the roof and there is the soft clatter of a bandicoot scurrying along the rafters. In the adjoining room, separated from this one only by a small corridor, coarse jute rope restrains a man to one of ten beds. He is screaming loudly in a psychotic rage induced by the atropine administered as an antidote to the insecticides he swallowed earlier today.

"Love problem, Doctor," Ramappa had told me earlier.

On another bed sits Shivarama, the other orderly, who has been assigned to watch over the restrained man.

The boy just sits there looking at the moths. Now Shivarama lights a leisurely *beedi*—an Indian hand-rolled cigarette—and watches us as we try to talk to the boy over the screams.

He tells us he is from a nearby village and has run away from home to the city after his stepmother beat him again for the fourth time this week.

I see bruises on his arms, his chest, and his back—black and red, they look like he has been playing *Holi*—the festival where people throw colored powders on each other to celebrate the first day of harvest season.

"I have sugar problem, Doctor," he says. The intern tells me to take care of this and goes to the next cubicle; another man has just been carried in after being hit by a speeding truck.

"I was taking injections for high sugar in my blood," he continues in fluent Hindi, "and then my mother died two months ago and my father married again. She has two children, so there is no money for injections now." He looks vacantly at the red-oxide floor. "I have been vomiting the whole day, Doctor, and now I feel like I will faint."

I examine him gently, afraid to push and prod too hard, his bones seem fragile and brittle with malnutrition. I feel his pulse—it is rapid and thready. His mouth is parched and he has the sick sweet breath of diabetic ketoacidosis.

"Do you get enough food to eat?" I ask.

"She says it is better to keep the food for healthy children, Sir. So my stepbrother and stepsister get most of the food. Anyway, it will be all wasted if I eat because very soon I will die from sugar disease."

As I examine him, I ask him how old he is.

"Eighteen," he says.

The fountain of youth for this boy is disease and malnutrition; his growth stunted and his development arrested, he looks about twelve.

I check his blood sugar. It is 664. I cannot check his electrolytes because the lab has run out of supplies tonight. "My sugar is high, no?" He looks at me. "If I did not have the disease, I could drink sweet, sweet juice every day—isn't it so, Doctor? My mother used to give me the juice of fresh oranges sometimes, before she died …"

I nod absently, worried about his condition. He is obviously in urgent need of fluids and insulin. "I am going to take him to the ward to get him admitted," I call out to the intern. There is no one to help us with a stretcher so we walk to the adult ward, the boy shuffling next to me in exhaustion and thirst. When we get to the ward, the clerk tells me the ward is full. I can see, over his shoulder, people crammed into every available bed, some accommodated on mattresses in the narrow corridors.

I decide to take the boy to the pediatrics ward. "Say you are sixteen," I tell the boy. I know admission criteria are strictly enforced and only patients under eighteen years of age are admitted.

"How old are you?" the admissions clerk asks the boy.

"He is sixteen," I tell the clerk.

"No, I want the boy to tell." The clerk glares at me, then turns to the boy again. "How old are you, I say?"

"Uh ..." His big black eyes are wide with nervousness and fear of this big-city clerk and big strange hospital building.

"Answer my question, I say!" the clerk points a pen at the boy, irritated by this delay in the proceedings.

"I am eighteen, Sir," the boy says softly.

"Then no admission. Sorry, Doctor, you are bringing adult person here. We can't admit him. He is adult," the clerk says pointing the pen at the boy again.

I know that here, in these aging government hospitals that take care of India's poor, bureaucracy reigns supreme. But I am angry with the clerk for enforcing petty rules when someone's life is at stake.

"Listen here, this boy needs treatment soon, otherwise he will definitely die. There is no place in the adult ward and that's why I brought him here."

But the clerk shakes his head again. "No, no admission here, he is adult."

"I don't care if he is an adult!" I say, feeling frustrated and powerless. "If you don't admit him I will speak to the medical superintendent and tell him that you denied admission to a critically ill patient."

"You can speak to medical superintendent, he will say the same thing," the clerk shrugs. "Either the boy will die, Sir, or if I admit him then the next child will die because we won't have any place in wards." He looks at the boy a little more sympathetically. "What can I say, Doctor, there are always more people than beds here. Sorry."

We walk back in silence toward the casualty, which is near the main gate of the hospital. The long, paved road is quiet, the darkness punctuated by soft lamps on the side. There are occasional sounds of crows; they are waking up, and soon it will be morning. The boy walks slowly, not talking, now and then wiping snot from his nose with a sleeve of his long ragged cotton shirt.

When we get to the gate, I hand him all the money I have in my pocket—50 rupees—about $1. He knows this will be enough only for a day's supply of insulin, but his eyes light up and he takes the money with a soft "thank you."

There is nothing else I can do. I watch him make his way through the big iron gates, past the waiting rickshaws outside. He waits for a bus to lumber past and then carefully, painfully, crosses the road. I watch him until he disappears into the shadows.

I feel sad and dejected, and this surprises me. I see disease and suffering all the time; every day people die for lack of money for medicines and tests. So this unaccustomed sorrow feels strange, but, like a long forgotten blanket, it begins to comfort me. Any feeling, even sorrow, is a respite from the numbness I wasn't even aware of until today. Then I realize that the soothing warmth of my sadness comes from this boy's despair. The selfishness of this confuses and disconcerts me, so I put it out of my mind and head back to the room to get some sleep before Ramappa knocks on the door again.

Later that day a body is brought to the morgue by a constable.

"We found him outside lying in the gully, Sir. It seems he drank many glasses of juice in that shop outside. Where he got the money from, I don't know, poor beggar."

I look at the boy. His legs are still scarred and his body is still bruised, but with his eyes closed and the smell of oranges clinging to him, he seems, finally, at peace.

*   *   *

Now I sit in this air-conditioned ward next to shiny computers and smooth new tables. I try not to think of the boy as I order this test for a 92-year-old woman with a dying mind and a dying body, a $2000 test that would buy lots and lots of insulin.

Medicine—Why I Left You

BEATRIZ M. RODRIGUEZ, MD

I left you because you left me first
I left you because I found you in bed with another
I left you because I could no longer find the good
people with whom I shared cadavers
I left you because you lied to me
You said you would never let business come in the way of
Our love
I left you because you made love to corporate America
I left you because you mistook ethics for the appearance of ethics
I left you because you lost control of yourself
Dining with CEOs and CFOs and market share
I left you because you looked me in the eye and said I don't
care what you think; I care only for what I need
I need to grow fat and I need to look good, I need to dominate
I need to feed the unquenchable desire of the market
I need to give people what they want not necessarily what they
need.
I need to pander
I need to be liked
I left you because you forgot who I was

You forgot that I had devoted my life to you
That I had sacrificed for you
That I stood in battle for you
That I defended you to the end
I left because I found you cared less for my
years of hard wrought experience than for
One MRI machine
I left because you asked spineless, blind men
to lead me and they defiled me
I left because my idealism was dying
I found that I had been chasing windmills
That I had believed the dream and it
was just that, a dream
And my heart was broken.
I left because you left me first.

Foreign Body of the Heart

LAWRENCE ZAROFF, MD, PhD

For doctors practicing for 20 to 30 years, the chance of avoiding a malpractice suit is equivalent to a tadpole growing wings and becoming a monarch. Theoretically, lawyers go after doctors only when medical care is not up to community standards. No lawyer, not even the most outrageous, would consider suing a doctor who lost a patient because of a stab wound to the heart—if the doctor and patient were on top of Mt. Everest. At 30 degrees below zero, wearing three layers of mitts, a skilled surgeon without equipment and anesthesiologist would be helpless. Not that a few lawyers—okay, a very few—wouldn't consider a lawsuit, whatever the circumstances, if they thought they could win a generous settlement.

For 29 years, I kept up with my changing specialty, asked for appropriate consultations, and was available when called, but a foreign body of the heart turned me into your average frog.

Mrs. Akin and her family were quietly pleasant when they appeared in my office for the preoperative examination and conference. A thin woman in her early fifties, she looked tired, wan. After her three children had grown, she had worked as a cashier in a convenience store until becoming incapacitated by fatigue and shortness of breath, evidence of heart failure secondary to calcific mitral valve stenosis and insufficiency. "Just glad to be in your capable hands" was her attitude as my explanations of the procedure and its possible complications evoked no questions.

Two weeks later, I replaced Mrs. Akin's diseased mitral valve with a mechanical prosthesis. The operation was without incident, easy, the diseased valve excised cleanly, and the artificial valve securely sewn in its place.

In operating rooms, counting is a virtue. Nurses account for everything; exactly the same numbers of sponges and instruments had better be there at the finish as at the start or the chest is not closed. If I quickly wired shut a sternum and a sponge was found to be missing, my insistence that their count was wrong was greeted with "Get an x-ray." And I always did. The counts for Mrs. Akin, however, were correct, and the postoperative course was uncomplicated. When I saw her two weeks after discharge, the incision was healing nicely, and she was significantly improved over her preoperative state, able to carry out her activities without symptoms. She was tearfully thankful.

*   *   *

He looked the part, a sly scowl, thin brush above narrow lip, tail hidden. What makes the messenger from hell smile when he hands you an announcement of a malpractice suit is proof of the man's pact with the devil. Especially when he knows that the cited amount is $10 million more than your insurance coverage. I felt like a Little Leaguer facing Randy Johnson—3 strikes and I was out. I was unaware of any fault; I was terrified; I knew that the whole damn thing was going to take a lot of time even if I eventually won. And finally I was furious. Before calling my malpractice carrier, I glanced at the main charge of the Akin's suit. Quite clear—I had left a foreign body in the lady's heart. Are there any more frightening moments than when you stand accused of a hurtful deed and have no idea how it happened? I turned to my operative note, which indeed stated that the sponge and instrument counts were correct. What was the foreign body?

Treading through the sludge in the legal document, I discovered that the accusation was based on a series of x-ray reports, which blandly and baldly pointed out, "The foreign body remains in the

[338]

heart." How did the lawyer get hold of these reports? I learned that the chart was never requested (the record room staff always notes chart movements). My unsupported speculation is that a kindly record-room clerk, while checking the chart for completeness, noticed the x-ray report and disclosed the misdeed.

I knew the resident who had read those chest films. He was a bit old to be a resident, having switched from the rigors of surgical training to the regular hours of radiology. Was this unconsciously an act of revenge against his former surgical oppressor? He understood my concern immediately and turned pale when the six chest x-rays of Mrs. Akin taken in the postoperative period were compared with the preoperative picture. All the postsurgical films showed the presence of an additional item. The foreign body, wedged between the left atrium and left ventricle, had not budged on the series of x-rays. Any first-year medical student would have known it was an artificial mitral valve. The resident should have reported, *The mitral valve prosthesis remains properly positioned between the left atrium and the left ventricle.* He took a shortcut. Nameless here but always to be remembered in the annals of cardiac surgery, the resident pleaded, "I was busy that month and just repeated the reading. I never thought that there might be someone, sometime, somewhere in the universe who would misinterpret." He deserved a splenectomy. I was restrained only by the knowledge I could easily abort the suit.

I remember every utterance of the next phone call. Few words, but each to Mrs. Akin's lawyer was delicious. He answered the phone, undoubtedly smiling at my opening remarks: "You are quite right. I did leave a foreign body in your client's heart." His response, incapable of restraint, was exuberant: "You admit you left something in Mrs. Akin's heart!" He was further heartened when I said, "Yes, but with another operation I could remove the foreign body." A pause for mental addition; then, "But, Doctor, that would cause Mrs. Akin a good deal of pain and suffering." When I interrupted his calculations to point out that the results of such an extirpation would cause more than pain and suffering, and might not be in Mrs. Akin's best interest, he became attentive. I heard his breathing. "Even a torturer can feel for his victim," I told him. Learning that the foreign body was her new valve, however, he could not disguise, did not try to, a groan, a sound a pig might make whose feed had been removed from his trough. "I hope you have not been too bothered, Doctor," were his final words. I did not nail him with, "Bothered? You jerk!" For all I know, this sudden reversal of his financial prospects may have killed him. Perhaps I should have dialed 911. Instead, my next call was to Mrs. Akin. When I relayed the same message to her, repeating the consequences of a second operation, I sensed she was going to have a chat with her attorney.

Bagatelle

CLAYTON J. BAKER, MD

No poet deserves praise
for remaining a poet.
Trifles stay trifles
however beautiful.
Floor sweepers, florists, fluoroscopists
win little acclaim
god knows, though god knows
a good verse
when (s)he hears one—
recalls her sun's gold reflection
in sparkling hardwood,
two dozen bloody bursting longstems or
the interlaced branching radiance of
this biliary tree silhouetted in
full intraoperative
bloom.

Sara and George and Justice

HOWARD FILLIT, MD

As an expert witness for the defense, I reviewed the case of a 90-year-old woman with Alzheimer disease who died of complications from a urinary tract infection in a nursing home. The case seemed like a typical clinical situation I had been involved with many times as a geriatrician, but in this case, the doctor was being sued for wrongful death.

Sara had lived in the nursing home for five years. George, her devoted husband, couldn't take care of her anymore. He put her in a "good home" and visited her every week, even as Sara became a nonverbal, completely dependent person with dementia.

George also picked a good doctor. Dr. H. ran an ethical, caring, competent practice. Dr. H. and George made a point of meeting at the home once a month. During the last year of Sara's life, Dr. H. and George had talked about advance directives. They agreed on a Do-Not-Resuscitate order, which was put in the chart along with documentation of the discussion itself.

After the umpteenth infection, George told Dr. H. that he did not want to hospitalize Sara anymore and would consider withholding antibiotics. George couldn't watch Sara suffer, and he knew Sara wouldn't have wanted this kind of life. George also told Dr. H. he had recently been diagnosed with lung cancer and that he was dying. He didn't want Sara to be alone, with nobody visiting or caring about her after he was gone. But after this long conversation, Dr. H. was in a hurry to get back to the office, and the discussion was not documented in the chart.

The following Friday night, Sara spiked a fever. Dr. H. told the nurse that it was probably another urinary tract infection and asked her to get a urine culture before he started antibiotics because it was probably a resistant organism. On Monday morning, Dr. H. called the nursing home, but the urine culture and sensitivity were still not back—a "problem with the lab." He told the nurse to call the lab and get the result, as was their usual practice, and to call him back.

By Monday night, the night nurse, who didn't know the case very well, got worried because Sara looked really bad. She tried to call George, but he was not available. The nurse decided that she needed to contact the next of kin, so she looked on the admitting sheet, made five years previously.

Sara was George's fifth wife. She was close to Betty, the daughter of George's third wife, so five years ago she, Sara, listed Betty as next of kin (and heir) after George. Unfortunately, soon after, George had a falling out with the family of his third wife. Betty hadn't seen Sara in five years and had not been involved in her care at all. However, the night nurse didn't know this and called Betty to tell her that Sara was looking really bad. Betty told the night nurse that she wanted Sara hospitalized immediately. The night nurse called Dr. H. and asked him what to do. He said that George's wishes were very clear, that Betty had not been involved in Sara's care at all, and that it was okay to keep Sara in the home. Again, he asked for the urine results, but again he was told they were not yet available. Tuesday morning, the results on the sensitivities were finally obtained, and Dr. H. started antibiotics. Sara died that afternoon, peacefully.

The reason the nursing home couldn't find George on that crucial Monday night was because he had been admitted to the hospital for exacerbation of his lung cancer. It also transpired that George had been having an affair for the past three years. Two weeks after Sara died, George remarried; at the age of 91, he took his sixth wife. Six weeks after Sara died, George died. The money in George's estate would now pass to his widow.

When Betty heard of George's death, she figured that if Sara's doctor had treated Sara aggressively, Sara might have lived longer than six weeks. George would then have predeceased her, his estate would have passed to Sara, and Sara's estate would have passed to Betty.

So, Betty sued Dr. H. for wrongful death.

We prepared to go to court. Dr. H. told me he could have settled out of court, even the insurance company wanted to, but he just couldn't admit to doing anything wrong after caring for Sara all those years.

We discussed his inconsistent palliative care plan. I asked him why he ordered the urine culture if he really wanted to withhold antibiotics. He said he hadn't quite formulated a clear plan by that Friday night, and that his first reaction was to do what he had always done with a urinary tract infection, to order the urine culture. He thought about starting empirical antibiotic therapy, but then he thought about George's wishes for palliative care, so maybe he decided to "go slow" and withhold the antibiotics until the sensitivities were back.

We tried to plan a strategy for the defense. I would testify about quality of life and the futility of treating recurrent urinary tract infections in patients with end-stage Alzheimer disease. However, I couldn't mention the last discussions that Dr. H. and George had about palliative care because they weren't documented in the chart.

In the back of the courtroom were Dr. H.'s wife and two little kids, there to support their dad on trial for wrongful death. The defense lawyer asked for my opinion. I testified that Dr. H. practiced within the standard of care. I tried to educate the jury about end-stage Alzheimer disease, but they were far away, across the room, across a chasm of knowledge and experience. I tried for over an hour to do my best teaching ever as a professor of geriatric medicine.

Now it was the plaintiff's lawyer's turn. I remember the patent leather shoes mostly. Handsome guy. Well spoken.

After about 90 minutes into testimony, he asked, "Shouldn't Dr. H. have gotten the urine results within 48 hours of the test, and was it not *his* responsibility to get the test results, not the nursing home's?" No, I said. While it was reasonable to get the results within 48 hours, it was Dr. H's practice to ask the nursing home staff to get the results, and the nurses blamed the delay on the lab.

Then he asked, "Doctor, in your expert opinion, if Dr. H. had treated the infection in a timely manner, would Sara have lived for 6 weeks, yes or no?"

I said I couldn't answer the question. Anyway, that was not the point. Alzheimer disease robs you of everything human. Treating the urinary tract infection was irrelevant and useless; antibiotics are futile at the end. Sara would have died of one of these infections whether they were treated or not. I couldn't mention George's wishes for palliative care, how maybe Dr. H. really wanted to withhold antibiotics in any case. But I gave my opinion that, for the values of most patients and their loved ones, this death was a blessing.

The judge let me go on (was he on my side?), despite the lawyer's objections. I was pleading with the jury, trying to convince them that Dr. H. provided compassionate, competent care. The lawyer finally demanded that the judge instruct me answer the question.

I said I thought it was unlikely that Sara would live 6 weeks, but that no physician can predict when death will occur with any certainty.

"So, it is *possible* then that Sara could have lived 6 weeks!? Yes or no?"

"Yes ..." There was nothing else I could say.

I left the courtroom thinking how unfair our tort system is. Dr. H. wasn't being judged by his peers. Three hours in a courtroom couldn't make the jurors understand, not medically, not emotionally, not ethically, what it meant to have end-stage Alzheimer disease. Because George wasn't there, nothing he had said about palliative care could be entered as testimony. This trial was all about money.

But for Dr. H., it was about his reputation, professional survival, and dignity. Accused in a small town of wrongful death of a 90-year-old nursing home resident! Dr. H. was a competent, caring physician, but he had an ambiguous, inconsistent palliative care plan. Nevertheless, in the end, he did carry out George's wishes. Sara did not suffer and died a peaceful death.

After a few hours the jury came back with a guilty verdict. Dr. H. was responsible for getting the results of the urine culture, they believed, and he could have started empirical antibiotic therapy. If he had, Sara probably would have lived six more weeks. Betty received $100,000. Dr. H. received a judgment for the wrongful death of a 90-year-old woman with end-stage Alzheimer disease, whose only loved-one sought compassionate care.

Justice was served.

After Insurance Issues
Are Settled

STEPHEN W. HWANG, MD, MPH

There's a new man here to see you," said Joyce, the nurse at the Toronto homeless shelter where I see patients once a week. "He just had his leg cut off. Says it hurts a lot."

I stepped out of my small examining room and into the hallway of the shelter. Micah was sitting quietly in a wheelchair, his pants already rolled up to reveal his right leg, which had been amputated below the knee. He was a brown-skinned man in his late 50s. He looked tired, and his black hair and mustache were streaked with advancing lines of gray. I introduced myself and asked him what the problem was.

"My leg's paining me again where they did the operation," he said. "And it's leaking." I rolled Micah into the examination room and removed the dressing covering his stump. The tattered gauze had not been changed since his discharge from the hospital 6 days ago, and it was soaked with a thin, yellowish fluid. The dressing emitted the unmistakable, nauseating odor of infection. A line of surgical staples surmounted the reddened and tender ridge of his wound, the edges of which were beginning to pull apart at one end.

Micah told me his story. Almost two decades ago, he had left his home in the Caribbean and had come to Canada on a temporary visitor's visa. He had stayed on since then, working full-time as a cook at a small restaurant and living in a basement apartment. He smoked cigarettes but didn't drink alcohol and had never used street drugs. About a year ago, Micah had noticed that he was thirsty all the time and went to see a doctor, who had diagnosed diabetes and prescribed him an oral hypoglycemic medication. The doctor's bill was not too bad, but the cost of the pills was more of a problem. After 3 months, Micah thought to himself, "Why am I buying this for so much money when I'm feeling okay?" He stopped taking the pills, and he never went back to see the doctor. (Canada has a system of universal health insurance that covers almost everyone, including most homeless people, but this coverage does not extend to undocumented workers.)

Two months ago, Micah's toes and then his entire right foot began to turn dark purple. After procrastinating for weeks, he finally sought care at the emergency department of a local hospital. By then, the gangrene was far advanced. Dr. Cabot, the admitting surgeon, had no choice but to amputate. Micah lost his apartment while he was in the hospital, as he had no income and little savings. In any case, access to his basement apartment had become impossible now that he was in a wheelchair. Homeless for the first time in his life, he had been discharged to the large downtown men's shelter in which we were presently sitting.

"When you were discharged, what arrangements did they make for your dressing changes and follow-up?" I asked Micah.

"Nothing," he said.

"Nothing?" I was both surprised and skeptical.

"They didn't give me nothing but this," he said, producing a neatly folded piece of paper. It was a hospital discharge form, the preprinted kind with spaces to fill and boxes to check. Under the section for "Follow-Up Appointments," the spaces for "Date" and "Time" had been left blank. In the area for "Comments," it read: "Follow-up with Dr. Cabot after insurance issues are settled."

I stared at the paper with a slight sense of shock. As an American trained in general internal medicine, I had seen many patients without health insurance who had delayed seeking care until their condition had become unbearable. Although I knew that uninsured patients might not be welcome at many hospitals and doctors' offices, it had not occurred to me that someone would have the temerity to tell a sick patient to stay away until he had insurance.

"Your leg has an infection," I told Micah. "You're going to have to go to the hospital right now to get it taken care of."

"Yeah, I was thinkin' that might be the problem," he replied calmly. I quickly wrote a brief note summarizing Micah's condition, while the staff at the shelter arranged for a taxi to take him to the emergency department of the hospital where I work, only a few blocks away.

Five hours later, I received a call from a somewhat irritated-sounding surgical resident. "We think it would be better if this gentleman were transferred back to the hospital where his original operation was done," he said. I told him that this would probably be difficult to arrange. "Okay, we'll see what we can do," came the reply.

The next morning, Joyce called to notify me that Micah was back at the shelter. The surgeons had performed an incision and drainage of his wound in the emergency department, prescribed oral antibiotics, made arrangements for regular dressing changes, and instructed him to return for follow-up in five days. Although Micah took the antibiotics faithfully, his infection worsened, and only two days later he had to be admitted to my hospital. He stayed for twelve days of intravenous antibiotics before returning to the shelter.

An orthopedic surgeon and an infectious disease specialist saw Micah once a month at the outpatient clinic of the hospital, a Catholic institution with a long-standing tradition of caring for the poor. I monitored Micah's progress during my weekly visits to the shelter. He took a prolonged course of oral antibiotics, and over the next two months his stump healed nicely. The shelter managed to arrange for the cost of his medications to be covered, and his diabetes came under reasonably good control. As his clinical condition stabilized, my encounters with Micah became less frequent. He moved into a smaller shelter, which provided him with some welcome relief from the noise and chaos of the shelter where we had first met.

A year has passed since Micah's amputation, and he is still homeless. Despite his situation, he is unfailingly pleasant and cheerful whenever I see him. He has not yet been fitted with a leg prosthesis because of his lack of insurance, but the staff at the shelter is trying to gather enough donations to buy one for him. Meanwhile, Micah gets around reasonably well in his wheelchair.

For people like Micah who lack health insurance, every illness—a nagging cough, a child with a high fever, the silent creep of diabetes—presents a wrenching dilemma: Seek treatment and face the resultant bills, or delay treatment and hope that the problem will take care of itself. As physicians, we eventually see the patients who have chosen the latter option when they have experienced a subsequent health catastrophe. However, we are insulated from the plight of the others who have made the decision to forgo health care. Perhaps they have heeded a clear, although unspoken, message: Our care is reserved for only those who can afford it.

The Cost of Doing Business

BONNIE SALOMON, MD

What's his insurance?
The psychiatrist on the cell phone demands.
Don't know, the hassled ER doc answers.
Oh, she knows.
She knows no form letter, shined shoe company
Would ever look at this
Homeless, hobbling schizophrenic, eyes wild,
Head on fire with delusions.

Last name, first name, middle.
He couldn't get past the first line.
Emergency contact—
The crack addict across the bridge.
Previous employers—
When he was 16, he loaded boxes
At Green's department store,
Fired when the voice told him to
Run into the street, losing a foot to a speeding truck.
Gross income—the four furry LifeSavers in a back pocket,
The three Sports Illustrateds found in the alley.

Magazines as amulets from the
Great Death the voice threatens.
Newsweek protects against pestilence, Life saves
His heart from stopping.

A mad underwriter might grant his petition.
An insurance company hearing a roar of voices
Shouting—
He's an excellent risk, actuarily sound: psychotic, perfect.
All premiums paid in full.

Sign him up.

On the Road

NANCY L. GREENGOLD, MD, MBA

Beanie Baby toys were selling for $5.95 at the hotel gift shop where I had just checked in. A customer was pawing through the koala bears, giraffes, and monkeys. "Ooh," she cooed, "You have cocker spaniels; I've been looking everywhere for cocker spaniels!"

"Those are $12.95," said the cashier, ringing up my Diet Coke.

"But they're smaller than the kangaroos—are you sure they cost more?" pleaded the Beanie Baby aficionado.

"Yep. Those are cocker spaniels. Everybody wants a cocker spaniel."

"Excuse me," I interjected, "is there an exercise room in the hotel? I just got off the plane from Los Angeles and I feel like a slug."

"Of course we have a fitness facility," she retorted. "Fifteen dollars a day, with a towel. But the pool's free."

"Darn," I said. "I didn't bring a bathing suit. And I only stair-step for about 10 minutes. Can I slip in for free?"

"Nope," said the cashier emphatically. "Nobody brings a bathing suit here; that's why the pool's free. Fifteen dollars a day for everybody, but you can spend the whole day if you like."

"Any place to stretch my legs around here?" I rejoined, thinking it must at least be free to take a walk.

"Oh, no," said the cashier. "Nobody walks around Chicago in January. You can't go out. Call the concierge and he will arrange transportation to the local mall. Everybody calls the concierge and goes to the local mall."

"Thanks a lot," I said. I would go instead to my room and download my e-mail and, as always, dutifully check my voice mail to learn what new "emergency" consultations in health services research required my presence. Perhaps there would be a stat managed care talk to give to some medical staff in Atlanta, or an urgent cut-costs-while-improving-quality meeting back home. The front-line physicians in the audience knew the lean/mean message was being cooked by the accountants, but we research types were supposed to make it more palatable by adding a dash of clinical acumen and a pinch of outcomes analysis to the stew.

I used to sit unnoticed in our hospital's doctors' lounge, listening to one after another physician lament his loss of professional control as well as the diminishing number of bagels in the lounge. They talked contemptuously of physicians like me—the "sell-outs" who had traded in their shingles for business cards. Except for my paltry 4 hours per week of "urgent" patient care, I had joined the enemy gurus of cost-containment. I represented "cookbook" and one-size-fits-all medicine, even though my spiel promoted evidence-based, blend-art-with-science, write-your-own guidelines.

In my presentations to our medical staff, I'd tried to bridge the gap between the administrators, with their disdain for arrogant docs who couldn't read a balance sheet, and the physicians, with their contempt for the fat-cat bean-counters who had never felt a spleen. Neither fish nor fowl, I was tolerated but not loved by any of them. My few weekly patients liked my bedside manner but were frustrated by my inaccessibility. Physicians who had admired me during training couldn't figure out why I was doing what I was doing, and thought it was a waste. The corporate types used me as medical window dressing but didn't especially want me in their board room.

I still wanted to act like a physician. I tried not to preach and did my best to listen. But the temptation to move up the proverbial executive ladder, to talk the predictable talk, to do what everybody else did to succeed, changed me nonetheless. I bought my carry-on with wheels. I got my laptop. I wangled airline upgrade certificates. And I took the evidence-based show on the road. And in short order, the job offers came flooding in. Yesterday a headhunter called, dangling an enormous salary in front of me for a medical director position at a large company in Columbus. I kept stammering, "Co-lum-bus?"

And he kept seducing, " Bonus ... stock options ... relocation."

"But what does the medical director *do?*" I kept asking.

"It's a top corporate position, reporting to the head of human resources. People would kill for a job like this." *Job like this.* When I demurred, unable to imagine anything more empty, he urged, "You can reach the highest level if you stay corporate. You'll move and shake with the best of 'em, and really end up running medicine. Better to rule than be ruled. *Everybody wants a job like this.*"

I thought of the corporate office with its corner window. Everybody should want a corner window. I thought of the company car and the frequent flier miles. I thought of the expense account and the schmoozy dinners. Everyone loves squid and shark and snails—the lower the phylum the better. What was wrong with me?

Police work was what stuck in my craw. Did I go through medical school, residency, and fellowship to be a cop? Better a copper than a coppee? No way, either way. As for the modern-day big-city doctoring job alternative, this was no loved and beloved Norman Rockwell house-call career, either. I thought of the bottomless pool of referral forms, the payment denials, the utilization review phone calls questioning my decisions. I thought of the missing-in-action medical charts, the lost laboratory tests, and the nursing assistants busy elsewhere whenever I truly needed them. I thought of the constant defensive documentation, of spending more time with paper than with people. I thought of the HEDIS measures, the physician report cards, and the knowledge that the national standard of "quality" I would have to meet had nothing to do with touching people, listening to their stories, and responding to their distress in any but a formulaic manner.

Which world was I to join? Full-time physicianhood would be true to my original dream but would lead to some embittering contemporary realities; the administrator role would leave me on the sidelines of medicine but with the illusion of control.

I returned to the gift shop and the land of Beanie Babies. I would be visiting my 9-year-old niece in a week, and I had to get her a gift. Everybody brings gifts to nieces. I wondered if she liked Beanie Babies. Didn't Shawna like kangaroos? I seemed to remember that she liked kangaroos. They were so tall, and they looked like $12.95 gifts. Three cute cocker spaniels surrounded one oblong kangaroo.

"All the kids like cocker spaniels," the cashier informed me as I reached for the kangaroo.

"Yeah," I countered, "but the kangaroo even has an extra head in its pouch. Isn't that more cost-effective?"

"Nope," the cashier snapped, "kids don't care much for kangaroos. Cocker spaniels are *in*. Everybody wants a cocker spaniel Beanie Baby."

I fumbled with my wallet, considering the cocker spaniels. They looked back at me, brandishing their identical, confident smiles. I didn't want to be cheap where Shawna was concerned. Maybe she would prefer a cocker spaniel, maybe she would consider it cool. I thought again of the medical director job in Columbus and knew that many of my peers would envy me if I took it. Most everybody wants a high-paying medical director job. I thought of the organization charts and the fitted suits. I thought of the strategic planning meetings, the P&L statements, the annual budget process—the making mountains out of a hill of beans.

In a moment of madcap independence, and to the chagrin of the cashier, I bought the kangaroo, buttoned up my unfashionable coat, and went out for a walk in the dirty snow.

HUP 2,3,4

ANNE E. HILLS

The peep-peep-peep from the hallway
is not a fluffy chick, under incubator,
but some measure of infusion or rhythm
holding the line between earth and heaven's reward (so, is earth a
    punishment?).
The hiss of air from the room vents is its accompaniment
never skipping a beat, supporting the concerto with soothing
    constancy.
I have been here through far too many movements with not a break
    for applause.
Across the street, Franklin Field stands guard under the overly moist
    skies.
Graduation day.
Wet, black gowns marking an end and beginning.
The cheering section went home before visiting hours were over.
Medicine is as relentless as loneliness.

Now, the darkness and I are left
to squabble over pointless things.

A Tale of Two Patients

FAITH T. FITZGERALD, MD

Late last year, my 87-year-old mother developed diarrhea. I phoned her doctor's clinic and was answered by a recorded voice that periodically told me, "All of our representatives are busy helping other clients. We appreciate your patience. Your call is important to us. Please hold for our next available representative." Synthetic music alternated with synthetic messages for 28 minutes before I lost my appreciated patience and hung up. I phoned again later; after a 15-minute hold, in the midst of "Your call is important …," I was disconnected. I got through on the third try. The first possible appointment was in two weeks. I took it. I would cancel my own workday afternoon to take my mother to see her doctor.

The receptionist ignored us when we came into the office at 3 p.m. I stood by her desk, Mom beside me in a wheelchair, while she chatted and joked with the clerk next to her for several minutes. I coughed. Nothing. I coughed more loudly. She glanced in my direction, so I quickly told her we were there for a 3:30 appointment. "Name?" she said. Then, "Registration card?" and "Insurance card?" She stamped a bunch of sheets of paper, then shoved a clipboard covered with a sheaf of documents to be signed toward me. We were directed to sit in the crowded waiting room. When we were settled there, I started to read the forms to Mom, but they were dense and in microprint, and largely unintelligible, so she finally just signed them unread. I carried them back to the clerk, who took them without a word. We waited some more. At 4 o'clock I went back to the desk. I stood in line behind more recently arrived patients and gradually worked my way to the front: "When will my mother be seen?" I asked the clerk.

"Name?" she asked. I told her. "Registration card? Insurance …?"

"We've done all that already," I said.

"Oh!" She shuffled though a pile of stamped papers, found Mom's, then put them back in the pile.

"Doctor is running behind. He'll see her as soon as he can," she said.

"Does he know we're here?"

"He'll see her as soon as he can," she repeated. She sounded annoyed.

"She feels miserable and tired," I said.

Even as I spoke, the receptionist picked up the ringing telephone and began to talk to the caller, turning her eyes away from me. I stood firm in my spot.

"Hey!" I said. She ignored me. "Hello! I'm still here."

"Excuse me," she said to the caller, putting her hand over the receiver. Then to me she said: "I'm on the phone!"

"I know that," I said. "When will my mother be seen?" It was now 4:15.

"Doctor will see her as soon as he can," she said, and resumed her telephone conversation.

I didn't move. When she hung up the phone, she looked around me to the next person in line behind me. "Name?" she asked him. "Registration card?"

I went back to my mother, who was sitting in her wheelchair holding her head in her hands. "Is the doctor going to see me soon?"

"He's running behind," I said.

"Does he know we're here?"

"I don't know."

"I'm really tired," she said.

"I know."

"What time is it?"

"4:20."

"Wasn't the appointment for 3:30?"

"Yes."

"Where is he?"

"Busy."

"I'm really tired," she said. "And I have to go to the bathroom."

"I'll take you."

"No. The doctor might come and not find us."

"I'll tell the receptionist where we are."

"No. I'm afraid we'll miss him."

"Do you want to go home? I can make another appointment."

"No. I'll wait."

Periodically, a nurse would come out of the inner office with a sheet of paper and call out a first name. "Bill?" she'd say, and a distinguished elderly man would get up. Then, 15 minutes later, "Harriet?" A woman stirred from her corner. Each time, my mother's hopes visibly rose with the nurse's appearance, then fell again, and she slumped back into her wheelchair when the name called was not hers. Finally: "Irene?"

I pushed my mother's wheelchair to the door. I said to the nurse. "My mother is 86 years old and from a time and place that equates respect with titles. Please don't call her by her first name."

Okay," she said, startled. "What shall I call her, then?"

I told her.

We were put into a cubicle. Mom's blood pressure, pulse, and temperature were taken. She was weighed, with great difficulty because of her immobility (I held her up on the small platform of the standing scales), and her body mass index was calculated from a wall chart. We were directed to an examination room that barely accommodated her wheelchair. It was cold. I asked the nurse for a blanket for Mom. She gave me a sheet. "We don't have any blankets," she said.

It was 5:30. "Is the doctor coming soon?" my mother asked the nurse.

"He's running behind," she said. "He'll be here as soon as he can."

"I have to go to the bathroom," Mom said.

"The doctor may want a urine sample," she said. "Can you wait?"

"I can wait," she answered.

"I'll take you," I said, and, over her protests, did. On the way to the bathroom, we passed a conference room full of laughing staff. They were having chips, coffee, cake ... a party of some sort. We took a long time in the bathroom to get done. Maneuvering Mom in and out of the wheelchair onto the toilet isn't easy. When we came back to the room, she was frantic. "Did he come? Did we miss him?" Just then, the harried doctor came in. He was apologetic, pleasant, polite, attentive, and thorough. He took a careful history and did a directed physical examination. "Her examination is normal," he told me, then more loudly to her, "Your exam looks okay, but we should get some tests."

"Now?" she asked.

"No," he said. "It's too late. The clinic lab is closed."

"When?" she asked.

"We can draw the blood tests tomorrow."

"What do we do now?" she wanted to know.

"You go home and eat a liquid diet until we know what's going on."

"No medicine?" she asked.

"Not until we know what's going on," he said.

He turned to me. "I'll give you a stool cup and urine specimen cup. You can bring them to the lab when you bring her for the blood draw." It was clear that, though he knew I was a medical school professor and had a clinical, administrative, and teaching schedule of my own, this was quite secondary to the system's constraints. If we wanted this done, it had to be done this way.

We went home, arriving well after 7 o'clock, both exhausted. The next day, after my early morning hospital rounds and rescheduling my non–patient care appointments, I took her to the lab, where a single, haggard phlebotomist faced about twenty patients.

Her diarrhea continued until the study results came back negative, then gradually stopped. "Probably something she ate," her doctor said when I phoned him with the news.

The bill, when it came three months later, was for over $600, mostly paid by Medicare.

*   *   *

Late last year, my 10-year-old boy developed diarrhea. I phoned his doctor's office, and the receptionist answered within two rings of the telephone. I explained the problem, and she said, in a voice of concern: "Oh, goodness. You'd better bring him in. Can you come in about an hour?"

"Sorry," I said. "I have appointments myself until this afternoon."

"Well, how about early this evening? Five o'clock? Five-thirty? Or we could see him this weekend."

"Five-thirty today is good. I'll get a chance to swing by home and pick him up."

"See you then. Call if you can't make it."

It was a squeeze, but I managed to get away early from work and arrived at the doctor's office only ten minutes late. The receptionist looked happy to see me, greeting me by title and last name, and was similarly welcoming to the patient. He was glum and anxious, but she was sympathetic. Within three minutes of our arrival, he had been weighed (markedly obese, as before), and we were led into a cheery, warm examination room. Four minutes after that, the doctor came in.

She spoke first to him; "How are you doing?" she asked. Then, as he turned away from her, "You poor guy. You don't feel well at all, do you?" She ran her hand gently through his hair.

He didn't answer.

"What's the problem?" she asked me and smiled sweetly at him. "It seems he's not up to talking."

I explained. She quickly, but thoroughly, examined him. He squirmed, uncooperative. She didn't seem to mind. A stool sample obtained by rectal exam was sent immediately for microscopy. "We'd better check a few labs," she said. The blood was drawn there and then. By the time she'd finished, the stool report was ready. "No white cells, no blood, no ova or parasites," she said. "His abdominal exam is normal, but we can get an abdominal radiograph to check for partial obstruction or volvulus if you like."

"Okay."

She took him to the radiography suite down the hall and returned in ten minutes without him, but with his film in hand, showing it to me on the view box: "Negative," she said. "Perfectly normal. We're getting a urine sample now," she said. "Sometimes a urinary tract infection can do this."

The urine and just-drawn complete blood count results accompanied his return to the examination room five minutes later. All was normal. The liver and renal chemistries would take a little longer, and the doctor promised to call me with them in the morning.

By this time, he looked better. I noticed that they had cut his nails, which had been a little long, while he'd been in the radiography suite. I was given dietary instructions by his physician. "No further therapy was warranted," the doctor said, and we left. The visit, exam, labs, radiograph, pedicure, and advice had taken half an hour and cost $175. He was hungry again that night, and his doctor phoned me first thing next morning to ask how he was doing and to give me his lab results—all normal.

"Probably something he ate," the veterinarian said. "You know how dogs are, and Igor is particularly dedicated to eating anything he can get his muzzle around." She laughed. "But if it happens again, just call us."

About the Editors

CHRISTINE LAINE, MD, MPH, Senior Deputy Editor of *Annals of Internal Medicine*, is a clinician, researcher, and medical educator who has worked in medical journalism for more than a decade. After receiving an undergraduate degree in writing at Hamilton College, she completed medical school at State University of New York at Stony Brook, internal medicine residency training at New York Hospital Cornell University Medical College, and fellowship training in general internal medicine and clinical epidemiology at Beth Israel Hospital Harvard Medical School. Dr Laine received a master's degree in public health from Harvard University. She is a clinical associate professor at Jefferson Medical College in Philadelphia, where she practices and teaches internal medicine. Praised by former *Annals'* editor Frank Davidoff as "perhaps the finest young mind in medical journalism," Dr Laine, among her many editorial duties at the American College of Physicians, co-edits the "On Being a Doctor," "On Being a Patient," and "Ad Libitum" sections of *Annals*. The mother of two young children, she has been held up as a role model for women physicians everywhere.

MICHAEL A. LACOMBE, MD, MACP, has developed a career that blends writing with practicing medicine. He is a graduate of Harvard Medical School, has practiced medicine for over 30 years in rural Maine, and is former director of cardiology at Maine General Medical Center in Augusta. Dr LaCombe is co-editor of the "On Being a Doctor," "On Being a Patient," and "Ad Libitum" sections of *Annals of*

Internal Medicine. He has published a book of medical advice for a general audience, *Medicine Made Clear: House Calls from a Maine Country Doctor* (Dirigo Press, 1989), and contributed to a second (*Empathy and the Practice of Medicine: Beyond Pills and the Scalpel*, Yale University Press, 1993). He served as editor of the two previous *On Being a Doctor* compilations. His *Pocket Doctor* was published in 1996 and *Pocket Pediatrician* in 1997. *Doctors Afield*, also published by Yale University Press and to which he contributed, was published in 2000. A collection of his stories of medicine is forthcoming from the University of Maine Press and, for ACP Press, he will edit two anthologies—one of poetry, one of prose.